# dyslexia?
## assessing and
## reporting

# The Patoss Guide

# dyslexia?
## assessing and reporting

# The Patoss Guide

Edited by
Gill Backhouse & Kath Morris

Project Coordinator: Lynn Greenwold

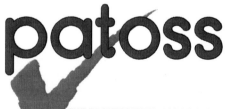

in association with

THE PROFESSIONAL ASSOCIATION
OF TEACHERS OF STUDENTS WITH
SPECIFIC LEARNING DIFFICULTIES

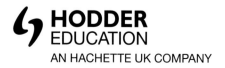
HODDER
EDUCATION
AN HACHETTE UK COMPANY

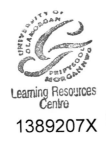
Although every effort has been made to ensure that website addresses are correct at time of going to press, Hodder Murray cannot be held responsible for the content of any website mentioned in this book. It is sometimes possible to find a relocated web page by typing in the address of the home page for a website in the URL window of your browser.

Hachette's policy is to use papers that are natural, renewable and recyclable products and made from wood grown in sustainable forests. The logging and manufacturing processes are expected to conform to the environmental regulations of the country of origin.

Orders: please contact Bookpoint Ltd, 130 Milton Park, Abingdon, Oxon OX14 4SB. Telephone: (44) 01235 827720. Fax: (44) 01235 400454. Lines are open from 9.00 to 5.00, Monday to Saturday, with a 24-hour message answering service. Visit our website at www.hoddereducation.co.uk.

A catalogue record for this title is available from the British Library.

ISBN 978 0 340 90019 2

First published in 2005 by Hodder Education, an Hachette UK company, 338 Euston Road, London NW1 3BH

Impression number     10
Year                              2012

Typeset in 11/13pt Stone Serif by Servis Filmsetting Ltd., Stockport, Cheshire

Printed in the UK by CPI Group (UK) Ltd, Croydon, CR0 4YY.

# Acknowledgements

As editors we wish to acknowledge the huge input made by the chief executive of Patoss, Lynn Greenwold. Lynn has coordinated the project from the beginning and has encouraged and cajoled contributors to ensure their chapters were delivered on time. She has been at the hub of our communications network. Although her name does not appear on the cover, she has been a more than equal partner in the editing process, where her wisdom, common sense and attention to detail have been invaluable. We hope that Patoss members will be among those who find this book useful and that Patoss itself will benefit from its association with this publication.

We have also appreciated the generous support of the late Oliver Backhouse, who spent a considerable amount of time formatting and collating chapters.

*Gill Backhouse*
*Kath Morris*

# The Editors

### Gill Backhouse

A Chartered Psychologist and Honorary Lecturer at University College, London, Gill assesses children and adults with literacy difficulties in an SpLD clinic there. She was formerly course tutor for OCR SpLD schemes at University College, London, and for three LEAs, and also an External and Chief Verifier for these schemes. Her previous publications are *The Patoss Practical Guide for Special Examination Arrangements* (two editions) and two chapters in Miles, T.R. and Westcombe, J. (Eds) (2001) *Music and Dyslexia: Opening New Doors,* London: Whurr Publishers.

### Kath Morris

Former scheme manager for OCR SpLD training schemes at Evesham College, Kath was an External and Assistant Chief Verifier for these schemes until 2004, and a member of the OCR working party which developed the new OCR suite of SpLD qualifications. An experienced learning support tutor, responsible for many years for carrying out diagnostic assessments both at Evesham and at North East Worcestershire Colleges, Kath is a founder member and former Chairman of Patoss.

# The Contributors

### Margaret Bevan

Co-founder of Partners in Education UK Ltd; develops and delivers SpLD training courses throughout the country and abroad.

### Valerie Hammond

Co-founder of Partners in Education UK Ltd; develops and delivers SpLD training courses throughout the country and abroad.

### Sue Kime

Senior Lecturer at the Centre for Special Needs Education and Research, University College, Northampton. OCR External Verifier for SpLD courses.

### Katherine Kindersley

Director of the Dyslexia Teaching Centre, London W8. Dyslexia Consultant to The Royal College of Art, Royal College of Music, Royal Academy of Dramatic Art.

### Bernadette McLean

Academic Director, Helen Arkell Dyslexia Centre. External Verifier and Examiner for OCR SpLD courses. Member of DfES working party on assessment of dyslexia in Higher Education. Co-author of Helen Arkell Spelling Test.

**Anne Mitchell**
Director of Services, Helen Arkell Dyslexia Centre. Member of the OCR working party formulating new SpLD qualifications and the DfES working party on assessment of dyslexia in Higher Education.

**Nick Peacey**
Coordinator of the Special Educational Needs Joint Initiative for Training, Institute of Education, University of London. Formerly Principal Manager for Equal Opportunities and Access at QCA.

**Prue Ruback**
Senior Lecturer in Primary Education at the University of Hertfordshire. OCR Chief Verifier for SpLD from 1996 to 1999.

**Liz Waine**
Senior Lecturer in Centre for Special Needs Education and Research at University College, Northampton. OCR Chief Coordinator for SpLD schemes. Member of the OCR working party for development of the new SpLD qualifications.

**Jennifer Watson**
External Verifier for OCR SpLD qualifications. Course Tutor and former Course Coordinator for OCR SpLD qualifications in Newcastle upon Tyne.

**Annie White**
Tutor and former scheme manager on the OCR courses in SpLD at Evesham College. Co-author of the successful teaching handbook *How Dyslexics Learn – Grasping the Nettle*.

# Contents

# Introduction

The aim of this book is to reflect the best practice of teachers and related professionals who assess learners for Specific Learning Difficulties from the early years to further and higher education.

The editors, as former chief and assistant chief verifiers for the OCR (formerly RSA) Specific Learning Difficulties schemes, were responsible for many years for moderating the standard of diagnostic assessments and reports produced by students. It was a time when understanding of dyslexia and other learning difficulties grew significantly. This was reflected in the growing availability of resources for assessment as well as teaching. Candidates on OCR courses had no difficulty in finding information from both books and the Internet for their Diploma essays, which almost invariably provided evidence of careful investigation and perceptive insight. However, the same candidates had more trouble in knowing how to complete their diagnostic assessments and reports.

It became clear, through the experience of verifiers and colleagues in teacher training, that a basic textbook on assessment for Specialist Teachers was needed. This book owes everything to the contributors, many of whom are course tutors as well as practitioners. They have willingly shared their experience in order to put good practice into a resource available to all those wanting to learn the skills involved in assessment. Each contributor, however, would gladly acknowledge how much they have learned from colleagues, students, tutors and especially from the children and adults whom they have assessed.

It was clear from the success of the Patoss guide on assessment for Special Examination Arrangements (Backhouse 2000) that Patoss could usefully play a role in promoting a book on a wider range of assessment issues for Specific Learning Difficulties.

Awareness of disability and its effects on education has grown in the past decade. Legislation such as the Disability Discrimination Act (1995) imposes a statutory duty on schools and colleges to ensure that pupils/students with a disability are not put at a disadvantage. To that end, assessment is a key tool in determining a person's individual strengths and difficulties and in planning appropriate support where necessary. Because of the demand for assessment, specialist teachers and SENCOs may now be required to fill a role which was once the province of educational psychologists. The training they receive must reflect this and ensure that assessment itself matches the need for the fair and equal provision that is required by legislation.

Initial training in understanding specific learning difficulties is important. Continued professional development is equally important. This book is therefore aimed both at teachers in training and those who wish to update their skills and knowledge. Just as this book will need revision to keep pace with the ever-changing society in which we live, so will the knowledge and experience of those who read it. Nothing ever stands still.

Dyslexia is just one of many learning difficulties, but it severely affects four per cent of the population. That is 80 students in a comprehensive school of 2000 pupils – a large number of people to be considered. We have concentrated on literacy rather than numeracy, but the recommended approaches may well raise concerns about other learning difficulties such as specific language impairment, dyspraxia (DCD), attention deficit hyperactivity disorder (ADHD), dyscalculia . . . . As we have compiled the book, we have realised how impossible it is to cover everything.

We hope that the way the book is arranged will satisfy readers who like a straight read from beginning to end and those who like to dip into chapters as they feel the need. To ease readability we have used the following gender conventions: teachers/tutors are female, learners are male. The book is in four parts. The first deals with the purpose of assessment and discusses the principles and practical aspects that apply to all age groups. The second focuses on how these apply to particular age ranges: foundation, primary, secondary, further and higher education. The third part considers the important issue of communication and partnership with others. The final section provides a straightforward guide to the psychometric principles underlying choosing tests and interpreting scores, the legal issues that are relevant to assessment, references as well as other useful resources.

Although the purposes of assessment may vary, the principles of good practice remain constant. Assessment should always promote a positive outcome and **never** be limited to discovering and labelling 'failings'. As long ago as 1968, Ausubel pointed out:

> *The most important single factor influencing learning is what the learner already knows.*

This is just as true today. Find it and teach accordingly.

*Gill Backhouse*
*Kath Morris*

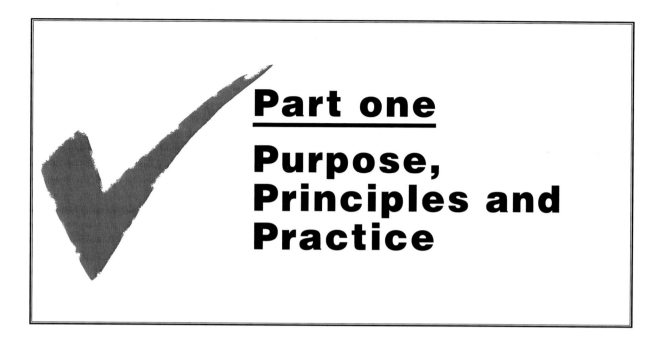

# Part one

# Purpose, Principles and Practice

# 1 The Purpose of Assessment

Kath Morris

'Where shall I begin, please, your Majesty?'

'Begin at the beginning,' the King said, gravely, 'and go on till you come to the end: then stop.'

(Lewis Carroll, *Alice's Adventures in Wonderland*)

In this chapter we shall begin at the beginning by considering why an assessment might take place, some of its specific purposes and some of the people and agencies that might be involved.

# What is assessment?

Various analogies have been used to describe assessment. Turner (1997) talks about testing in terms of an experiment where we are not sure of the outcome – there is the possibility of learning something new. An assessment also might be compared to a detective story where we search for evidence in order to uncover more of the truth, or even a jigsaw puzzle where pieces are fitted together to create a picture. All of these are useful analogies, but cast the learner – the person being assessed – in a passive role.

We would like to stress the interactive nature of assessment as a process where learners are very actively involved – in completing tests, but equally importantly in talking about and demonstrating the ways they learn best, their coping strategies, their motivation, their interests and their goals. Another important kind of interaction is that between the assessor and other interested parties – fellow professionals, parents, carers and possibly employers. Many people and agencies might be involved. Assessment is not therefore an isolated event, but part of an interactive process whose purpose is to understand a learner better and to promote his best interests.

# Why assess?

## To address concerns and identify needs

Although every learner has a different set of circumstances, there are common themes which often come to light when we look at the route which has led to an assessment. First and most obvious of these is concern about educational progress. In the case of children, it is very often parents or carers who seek an assessment, either privately or through the school system, because they feel that their child is failing to make progress as expected. A suspicion that dyslexia might be a reason for this might be prompted by family incidence of dyslexia. Family history is not a *cause* of dyslexia, although we have seen this written into some reports. It is certainly a risk factor.

With no family incidence, parents might not be so alert to the possibility of dyslexia. However, knowledge about the condition and access to information is now much more widespread than it was even ten years ago, through schools, books, magazine articles, TV, radio and local dyslexia groups. Mothers are very often well informed as to what to look out for. In their observations of their child's progress, they are only too aware of any differences which might indicate that the child does not fit quite happily into the normal educational pattern and may be, even at a young age, showing a different approach to learning. A mother's observations of her child's development are always important. It is worth noting here that whilst we know that the cognitive difficulties associated with dyslexia can occur across the ability range, they are more obvious in a child who seems to have good cognitive abilities but does not progress in language and literacy skills.

Teachers and teaching assistants involved in pre-school and early education are also alert to possibilities of learning difficulties. For learning difficulties and/or disabilities which cause serious concern, even in pre-school the Special Educational Needs Code of Practice (2001) defines Early Learning Action and Action Plus. At this stage, difficulties in acquiring speech could be one reason for action and possibly for referral to a speech and language therapist. However, for learners with dyslexia, more formal systems are likely to come into play later, when teaching of literacy and numeracy skills becomes more central to the curriculum. Children who have difficulties in acquiring these skills might not progress as expected, despite the additional learning support which is usually provided in groups. At this point, an in-depth individual assessment might be thought necessary, particularly if a screening package such as the **Dyslexia Screening Test** or **CoPS** (Cognitive Profiling System) has indicated a risk of dyslexia.

At a later stage in education, concerns might change and need to be addressed in a different way. It is often the case that whilst some students with dyslexia do well as they progress through secondary, further and/or higher education, for many the heavy demands on memory, the amount of planning and organisation involved and the sheer amount of coursework to be completed cause ever-increasing stress. Very often these students have not been identified as having any problems before. They may not be severely dyslexic but, as the demands of the curriculum have grown, their ability to cope has been put under more and more pressure. The same thing can happen in vocational training programmes and in employment, giving rise to concern not only from the individuals affected but also from those working with them.

## To diagnose difficulties and ascertain strengths

Whilst dyslexia might give cause for concern, many students, particularly adult students, are as much interested in finding out about themselves as they are concerned about their progress. This is also true of adults who are no longer in education. Very often the prompt comes from the fact that a parent whose child has been diagnosed as dyslexic recognises some of the child's strengths and difficulties as his own and requests an assessment.

Dyslexia is now usually considered as a continuum of difficulties, so that people can pass through the educational system – particularly if they have only slight difficulties – without being identified. Maybe they have always felt that some things that others managed easily were inexplicably hard for them – but at other things they showed surprising talent. An older generation of people was educated in the days when there was little or no recognition of dyslexia. They have often suffered a lifetime of frustration and misunderstanding.

It is very important for these people that the assessment clarifies the sorts of difficulties they have, explains how these are balanced by some often surprising strengths, and suggests some ways in which these strengths can be optimised. It should always be the aim for assessment to be a positive rather than a negative experience.

## To establish a level playing field

There are three main sources of support through the legal system available to disabled learners.

*1* Under the Disability Discrimination Act (1995), schools are required to provide protection for disabled children by preventing discrimination against them. This imposes two key duties on schools:

- not to treat disabled pupils less favourably;

- to take reasonable steps to avoid putting disabled pupils at a substantial disadvantage.

A disabled person is defined as someone '*who has a physical or mental impairment which has an effect on his or her ability to carry out normal day-to-day activities*' and covers any physical or mental disability, including sensory impairment and other 'hidden' disabilities such as mental illness, learning disability, dyslexia, diabetes and epilepsy.

2   The Special Educational Needs (SEN) Framework places duties on schools which are based on the definition of SEN in the Education Act 1996. This says that: '*A child has special educational needs if he or she has a learning difficulty that calls for special educational provision.*' The purpose of the SEN Framework is to make provision to meet the special educational needs of individual children.

3   The planning duties are contained within the Disability Discrimination Act and address three distinct areas of access: access to the curriculum, physical access to education and associated services, and the provision of information in a range of formats for disabled pupils.

The same principles underlie legislation affecting post-16 education.

One of the purposes of assessment in an educational context, therefore, might be to establish the extent of a learner's difficulties, the extent to which they disadvantage him and to advise how his special educational needs might be met. Similarly, in employment or training, an assessment might be called for with a broadly similar purpose.

A good example of this sort of assessment is the assessment for Disabled Students' Allowance (DSA). The initial assessment for this allowance may, in the case of dyslexic students, be carried out by an educational psychologist or appropriately qualified specialist teacher.

# To assess the need for special examination arrangements

Assessments for Access Arrangements in Examinations could be said to have the same purpose. They are sometimes misconstrued as conferring advantages. This should certainly not be the case. The purpose of an assessment decision to allow extra time, a reader, an amanuensis or other accommodation is not to make a dispensation or concession, but to allow each candidate equal opportunity to demonstrate his knowledge, understanding and skills without being disadvantaged by a disability. Whether this is a physical disability, sensory impairment or learning difficulty, the same principle applies. Quite complicated procedures are in place to prevent abuse of the system, and those carrying out this particular type of assessment must understand them.

The importance of being able to measure certain abilities, attainments and cognitive skills is particularly relevant to this purpose of assessment. Test scores provide the important quantitative evidence through which an individual's performance might be compared to others in the same age group. If the assessment is to have professional integrity, it is essential for assessors to understand how to score standardised tests correctly and to understand their meaning.

## To plan intervention

Very often specialist teachers (even experienced ones) who carry out assessments find it easier to come up with accurate scores and a sensitive and detailed description of a learner's strengths and weaknesses than to recommend appropriate intervention. Making recommendations and planning targets is not an easy thing to do well. However, it is no use diagnosing a problem without suggesting a remedy.

In most cases it will be very important for an assessment report to present plans for an appropriate teaching programme. It is important to say 'usually' here, as the sort of information needed by those requesting an assessment may vary. In many schools it may be that after an assessment a specialist teacher will go in to a school and initiate a consultation about teaching objectives and methods, rather than 'imposing' a teaching programme. It is almost always the case that the preferred method of accommodating a learner with dyslexia will be to promote a dyslexia-friendly learning environment as well as, or even instead of, plans for one-to-one intervention. However, training courses in assessment will want to see that candidates have the skills to plan for both classroom support and individual programmes.

## To review progress

Sometimes an assessment is required to review a learner's progress since a previous assessment. Specialist teachers may be asked to 'update' a report carried out previously, very often by an educational psychologist. Reports written more than two years ago will need to be updated if they are to be considered valid by exam boards.

# Who will read the report?

Many years ago, the phrase 'a sense of audience' began to be used widely to express the idea that writing was not just done in a void. It had to address a particular group of readers who were the intended audience. This phrase comes to mind when talking about the purposes of assessment – particularly when thinking about how the report should be slanted.

The purposes we have described are certainly not mutually exclusive: many will overlap. Nevertheless, purpose and intended audience will influence the way the assessment is conducted, the way the report is written, and the emphasis which is given to different pieces of information. This issue is about communication and will be considered in Part 3.

## Summary

- Assessment is an interactive process in which both the learner and the assessor are actively involved.
- There is also likely to be involvement from other interested parties – parents, carers, teachers, other professionals and sometimes employers.
- The individual learner is at the centre of the process.
- Assessments may be:
  1 to address concerns and identify needs;
  2 to recognise individual strengths and ways of working and to diagnose difficulties;
  3 to promote a level playing field;
  4 to assess the need for examination access arrangements;
  5 to plan intervention;
  6 to review progress.
- These purposes are not mutually exclusive, but will influence the way the assessment is conducted and the report written.

# 2 Principles of Assessment
## Gill Backhouse

'Too often examiners forget the dictum that "Tests don't diagnose, people do" and base their diagnoses exclusively on test results, a hazardous enterprise at best. Test results are merely observations, . . . but do not tell the examiner why a person performed as he or she did. . . . Test results make useful contributions to diagnosis, but in the end practical diagnoses rest on the clinical skills and experience of examiners.'

(Wagner, Torgesen and Rashotte 1999)

The clear message conveyed by this quotation is that the professional skills and judgement needed by competent assessors extend far beyond knowing which tests to use and how to interpret the results – important as these are. Knowledge of the normal development of literacy skills and the relevant underlying cognitive processes, plus the ability to recognise the signs of specific difficulties right across the age range, are all essential prerequisites for the skilled diagnostician. Furthermore, the ability to bring into the picture an understanding of environmental influences and the effects of educational experience (including remediation), as well as affective factors such as temperament and motivation, is vital when trying to determine the most probable cause(s) for any one individual's difficulties and the best way forward. Each time we test out a developing hypothesis of what the learner's underlying problem might be, our choice of tests becomes important. The skilled assessor needs a range of assessment resources with which to examine literacy skills in a comprehensive and relevant way and to probe various cognitive functions. The assessor's skills are immeasurably strengthened by the knowledge accrued from practical experience of teaching learners with and without literacy problems.

Before considering these various issues, we must not forget that children learn to speak long before they learn to read and write, and that literacy is in effect spoken language in code. The many facets of spoken language include:

■ knowing which sounds (**phonemes**), in which order, make a particular word (**phonology**);

■ the ability to produce the word (**articulation**);

■ knowing what words/phrases mean (**semantics**);

- knowing about grammar: word structure (**morphology**) and sentence structure (**syntax**);

- the use of language to communicate with others (**pragmatics**).

In all these respects, oral communication involves both **listening** (*reception*) and **speaking** (*expression*). Clearly any difficulties at any level with spoken language will be reflected in the acquisition and use of literacy skills.

Research into the normal development of reading and writing has largely been driven by the need to understand conditions such as dyslexia, which first becomes really apparent when children have inordinate difficulties with *cracking the code* and basic *word*-level skills. We need to understand what is required to take these first steps.

# Normal development of literacy skills: what is involved?

In English, we convert speech into written language using an alphabetic code – one or more symbols for each sound (phoneme) uttered.

The first task for beginners is to learn the basic code – sound-symbol correspondence. But when speaking English we actually use 44 sounds – 20 vowel and 24 consonant sounds.[1] The task of mapping 26 abstract shapes (letters) onto these is a huge one, not only for young minds, but on a continuing basis as spoken vocabulary and the use of different grammatical constructions expands.

Furthermore, English is an extremely **opaque** language in the sense that the relationship between speech sounds (phonology) and spelling patterns (orthography) is not reliable. There is one rule, however, that really works: there must be at least one vowel, or a *y*, in every syllable to represent the voiced and mouth-open sound at its heart. We have a great many exceptions or irregular words (*said, yacht,* etc). We also have to contend with homophones (such as *there/their/they're; bean/been*), whose correct spelling can only be deduced from the context of the word when the meaning is known. There is no doubt that the task of becoming a proficient reader and speller in English is much harder than in more **transparent** languages. For example, mapping letters onto speech sounds in Italian or Greek is a more straightforward affair (Goulandris 2002).

---

[1]  Vowel sounds are all voiced and made with the mouth open. Consonant sounds are voiced or unvoiced and the flow of air is obstructed using the tongue, teeth, lips.

Small wonder that the time taken for the majority to 'crack the code', as well as the incidence of severe dyslexia, is particularly high in English-speaking countries.

When learning to spell words we need to break up (**segment**) the word into its constituent sounds (*phonemes*) before we can apply our spelling (*orthographic*) knowledge. Research has shown that there is a developmental pattern regarding segmentation skills. Very young children are only able to identify fairly large 'chunks' of sound (*syllables*) and gradually become more discerning as awareness of alliteration and rhyme develops. In the early years at school their **phonological awareness** develops further as letter sounds are taught. As pupils learn to spell, they see patterns emerge as spellings are mapped onto sounds. When using phonics to decode a word, they need to **blend** sounds together and check whether they know such a word (lexical checking). Gradually, children learn to identify all the phonemes in words, including consonant blends. Unstressed sounds such as /*m*/ and /*n*/ in final blends (-*mp*, -*nd*) are generally the last to be differentiated.

How are these three issues – word-level reading and spelling, underpinned by phonological awareness – connected in a developmental framework? We need to have a good grasp of what normal development looks like before we can judge whether a learner's skills are age-appropriate in all respects, mildly delayed but following a normal pattern, or showing unusual signs as well as being delayed.

Frith (1985) developed a well-known model of the development of word-level reading and spelling skills. Although superseded by more complex phase models (Ehri 2002) as well as qualitatively different connectionist theories (Seidenberg 2002), Frith's model is easy to understand and apply and therefore recommended for everyday use in assessment (Figure 2.1).

**Logographic** reading is conceptualised as a visual strategy, a kind of look and guess based on partial visual cues. It is inaccurate and similar-looking words are muddled (e.g. *sleep/steep/sheep*). The child has no decoding skills, so cannot work out unfamiliar words.

**Alphabetic** skills develop as letter/sound knowledge grows and he 'cracks the code'. The child can now use sound-based strategies to decode and encode, so reading of unfamiliar words and spelling become possible. Emergent spelling clearly requires considerable phonological awareness, as well as sound-symbol correspondence.

**Orthographic** knowledge then needs to be consolidated. As reading experience and spelling instruction are integrated with semantic and grammatical knowledge, much word-specific, also 'sub-lexical' knowledge (applying to divisions within words) is acquired. Spelling rules, common spelling patterns (e.g. /-*tion*/, /-*een*/, /-*ed*/, /-*ing*/, irregular forms, homophones, etc) are mastered.

| Age | Reading | Spelling |
|---|---|---|
| | **Logographic**<br>Early reading is BY SIGHT.<br>Learning is by 'Look and say'.<br>New words cannot be read.<br>Similar looking words are muddled. | |
| | **Alphabetic**<br>Ability to work out new words<br>using phonics develops.<br>Sight vocabulary increases. | **Alphabetic**<br>Early spelling is BY SOUND.<br>Spelling is phonetic – i.e. it<br>sounds right.<br>(Awareness of sounds in<br>speech AND letter-sound<br>knowledge are necessary<br>pre-skills.) |
| | **Orthographic**<br>Fluent, accurate reading depends<br>on an amalgamation of visual<br>and phonic strategies. Attention<br>is paid to both the overall shape<br>*and* the internal structure of a<br>word. | **Orthographic**<br>Correct spelling develops as a<br>result of reading experience AND<br>spelling instruction, semantic<br>and syntactic knowledge. |

**Figure 2.1** A model of the normal development of (single-word) reading and spelling skills (Frith 1985)

A useful aspect of this model is that it offers an explanation of why children can often read words they cannot spell, and write words they cannot read. The hypothesis is that, in the early stages, they use different strategies for the two tasks: reading by sight, but spelling by sound. Then gradually the two processes start to interact, one feeding the other in a dynamic way. It follows, therefore, that early spelling ability will be a better predictor of reading progress than early 'logographic' reading success. It should be emphasised that these 'stages' are not seen as discrete phases that children move into at particular ages. Rather, the model represents a fluid process that is gradually worked through as the relevant strategies develop and word-specific knowledge is acquired.

From the assessment point of view, it offers a method of evaluating spelling mistakes to see if they appear 'acceptable' from a developmental perspective. If 'spelling by sound' is the norm, it follows that mis-spelled words should still reflect the sequence of sounds in the target word when it is spoken. The degree to which this is achieved will depend on the learner's segmentation skills and letter knowledge. Young children may well only use a few letters to represent the dominant sounds in a word (e.g. *lk* for *look*). As their knowledge of sound-symbol correspondence increases and they become more adept at 'sounding out', we see attempts such as *jupt* for *jumped* – but the hard to detect /m/ is not yet evident. Both these attempts are classified as **semi-phonetic**, since although not all phonemes are represented, those present are in the correct order. Spelling where at least one letter has been put down for every phoneme – *sed/said, pecos/because, rynoserus/rhinoceros* – is called **alphabetic spelling** for obvious reasons. Finally, when spelling is correct – that is, the specific patterns and rules of English have been absorbed – we say that full **orthographic** competence has been reached. According to this model **dysphonetic** spelling, where the sequence of letters does not reflect the order of sounds in the spoken word, would raise concerns.

Reading, however, is much more than recognising single words. Its purpose is to gain meaning from text. The skills required can be conceptualised as a combination of 'top-down' and 'bottom-up' processes. The top-down processes are those brought to the text and rooted in spoken language skills – vocabulary and grammatical knowledge, the ability to infer from context and predict what is coming next, the use of general knowledge to add to and/or check for meaning and sense. The bottom-up processes refer to the ability to decode the marks that are on the page. Effective top-down processes can compensate for weaker bottom-up skills and research has shown that good oral verbal skills help 'bootstrap' word recognition in dyslexic readers to a greater extent than in their non-dyslexic peers (Snowling 2000).

The equation developed by Gough and Tunmer (1986):

$$R = D \times C$$

where **R** = reading comprehension, **D** = decoding ability, **C** = linguistic comprehension, is a useful one to bear in mind. It emphasises the interdependence, when reading, of two independent variables: decoding skills and the ability to understand language.

Good decoding skills but poor receptive language skills may be seen in children with general learning difficulties; excellent listening comprehension but poor decoding skills in bright dyslexics. Neither will have good reading comprehension – particularly in the latter case, if speed is taken into account. Thus comparisons between listening and reading comprehension are of particular interest when identifying dyslexia.

# Dyslexia: definitions, signs and symptoms

At this point we have to acknowledge that there is no one universally agreed definition of **dyslexia**! All descriptions of this condition acknowledge the main problem as trouble with reading and spelling. However, a quick trawl through the literature will immediately reveal under this heading a whole host of other symptoms, including trouble with maths and personal organisation. Varied causes are also implicated relating to unusual patterns of activity in different areas of the brain – e.g. language areas, visual pathways or the cerebellum (DfES 2004a). A recent review of the literature concluded, perhaps controversially, that

' *Dyslexia is not one thing but many – to the extent that it may be a conceptual clearing house for a variety of difficulties with a variety of causes.* '

(Rice and Brooks 2004)

It is undeniable that many learners as well as their parents find a diagnostic label comforting and reassuring, and there are arguments both for and against labelling. One problem with labels, however, is that all too often we see aspects of several types of difficulty in the same learner (e.g. dyslexia *and* dyspraxia). In fact **co-morbidity** is often thought to be more common than 'pure' syndromes – always supposing that there is a consensus as to what constitutes a pure syndrome! Since definitions already vary and will no doubt change as the knowledge base increases over the years, a descriptive approach that specifies the problem is to be preferred. Probable cause(s) and recommendations slot neatly alongside this type of diagnosis, which is far more helpful than simply labelling learners as dyslexic. This is why the concept of **specific learning difficulties** is generally more useful and used as an 'umbrella' term for a wide range of learning difficulties, such as dyslexia, dyspraxia, dyscalculia, ADHD and so on.

The *Diagnostic and Statistical Manual IV* published by the American Psychiatric Association (APA 1994) defines specific learning difficulties in the following way:

- *'impaired ability to develop a skill (or set of skills) to an age-appropriate level or to a level consistent with other abilities;*

- *the difficulties interfere significantly with academic achievement or daily life;*

- *the problems are not caused by a medical condition;*

- *adequate opportunities to develop the skills have been available.'*

This is a very useful definition to keep in mind as it:

- enables learners of all levels of general ability to be included and invites one to compare and contrast strengths and weaknesses;

- suggests a meaningful way of quantifying the difficulties;

- excludes those whose problems stem from medical or environmental reasons and thus places the cause firmly in the cognitive domain.

However, *all* difficulties encountered by a learner during his education and training, whatever the causes, need to be addressed. This is nowhere more true than with regard to literacy skills – so fundamental to progress in all subjects right across the curriculum and age range.

The Division of Educational and Child Psychology of the British Psychological Society (BPS 1999) proposed a 'working' definition of dyslexia, which now forms the basis of much LEA policy. It acknowledges that all school children with intransigent literacy problems need help if they are to access the curriculum and states:

*Dyslexia is evident when accurate and fluent word reading and/or spelling develops very incompletely or with great difficulty. This focuses on literacy learning at the "word level" and implies that the problem is severe and persistent despite appropriate learning opportunities. It provides the basis for a staged process of assessment through teaching.*

Dyslexia is thus defined as a **primary** difficulty with reading and spelling **single words**: in learning and using the **coding** system for representing spoken words in their written form. It is the definition used throughout this book, but it does **not** include particular problems with fine motor skills and handwriting, or maths for example, although these are often associated with dyslexia. Furthermore, it does not specify the cause of such difficulties, although it suggests 'within child' (i.e. cognitive) factors, by requiring the trouble to be *severe and persistent despite appropriate learning opportunities.* Importantly, it emphasises that assessment should be ongoing and part of intervention: not only used to plan a support programme but also to monitor progress. We must also remember that a 'snapshot' taken at an individual, one-off assessment – pointedly referred to as 'dipstick testing' (Reason 2004) – although having many advantages, must not be taken as valid and relevant unless and until the results are considered in the context of the learner in his normal educational context.

The symptoms of dyslexia vary in a number of ways. The most obvious factor is age, and a **developmental perspective** is essential to our understanding. What starts out as a phonics/word-level problem, begins to look rather different as the dyslexic child grows older and acquires some basic skills. The 'knock on' effects of difficulty and delay in 'cracking the code' manifest themselves in diverse ways. Factors such as the general ability and motivation of the student, as well as the quality of his learning environment and availability of learning support, will all affect the outcome. Contributory causes may differ and compound each other. Chapters 4–7 all begin with an account of the range of problems typically seen in the different phases of education.

In the past, definitions of dyslexia usually excluded children of below-average IQ. This was because difficulties in acquiring age-appropriate literacy skills were seen as part and parcel of general learning difficulties. However, we now know that dyslexia affects people right across the ability range. Those with general learning difficulties can acquire reliable word-level skills, whereas some extremely able individuals appear unable to grasp and operate the same system with any degree of accuracy or fluency, no matter how hard they try. Why should this be? What has research uncovered about the differences between such individuals and those who do not have any literacy difficulties? An up-to-date understanding of the knowledge base will influence and inform assessment as well as teaching practice.

# Research during the last 25 years

We need to consider the way research projects are conducted to appreciate the reasons for different aspects of thorough assessment practice.

Many projects focus on groups matched for age and IQ (both children and adults) and look at the differences between good and poor readers in terms of the kind of words they have trouble with (e.g. regular or irregular), the type of spelling mistakes they make (e.g. 'near misses' or bizarre), and the integrity of their auditory, visual and memory processing.

Others studies compare groups of children with the same **reading age** and IQ – even though the 'dyslexics' are likely to be two or more years younger than the 'normals'. This excludes any differences stemming from reading experience.

A third line of enquiry has focused on the development of children's literacy and associated skills (including those deemed 'at risk' when they started school) by assessing the same children year on year. Some of these longitudinal studies have also compared children's responses to different methods of teaching reading and spelling (Hatcher 2000).

On a different tack, investigating the incidence of dyslexia in families has led to the understanding that there is a heritable predisposition to this condition. More recently a certainty that it is biologically based has grown from the use of brain-imaging techniques. These have shown functional differences between the brains of dyslexics and carefully matched controls, during language-based tasks.

The expanding interest in comparing dyslexia in different languages has opened up a rich seam of understanding concerning the importance of the linguistic environment.

It will be seen that these different approaches are focusing on very different issues – ranging from brain imaging to the nature of spelling mistakes. The importance of being aware of these differing levels of analysis was encapsulated in the well-known Causal Modelling Framework (Morton and Frith 1995) and is extremely helpful in the context of diagnostic assessment (Figure 2.2).

| | BRAIN (*the biological level*) |
| ENVIRONMENT | MIND (*the cognitive level*) |
| | BEHAVIOUR |

**Figure 2.2**  Causal modelling framework (Morton and Frith 1995)

The model encourages us to consider separately, the **biological** level (heritable, genetically based indicators), the **cognitive** level (the mental processes about which we hypothesise on the basis of our diagnostic tests and observations), and the **behavioural** level (the aspects of reading and writing which we can directly observe). **Environmental** influences (positive or negative) must also be taken into account at all three levels.

As the knowledge-base regarding literacy acquisition and dyslexia has increased enormously (although not yet complete), there is a wide consensus in one regard – that weaknesses in **phonological processing** are a major issue in dyslexia. This contrasts with notions of visual processing deficits, which held sway from the beginning of the twentieth century until about 1980. Then the link between literacy problems and language was perceived and 'word blindness' concepts gave way to linguistic deficiency theories. Subtle deficits in speech processing are now recognised as the defining features of developmental dyslexia. This is not to say that no other aspects of cognition are involved in the aetiology of literacy difficulties – but that at present, more is known and understood about **phonological deficit** theories than any others.

# Assessment: theory and practice

Let us now explore the phonological deficit in dyslexia at the four different levels set out in the causal model above and how such knowledge informs and structures our assessment procedures.

# Biological level

Since we know that dyslexia runs in families, a history of language/literacy problems within the family (e.g. parents, grandparents, siblings, cousins) places a child 'at risk' of similar difficulties.

As phonological processing is fundamental to the development of speech, the child with some degree of impairment in this regard may well exhibit typical signs pre-school. Delays in learning to talk; immaturity of speech and/or language skills prior to the onset of formal instruction in learning to read and write; referrals to Speech and Language Therapy pre-school are all 'at risk' factors.

■ Therefore, responses to well-constructed questionnaires (see page 183) focusing on family and developmental history are an important part of assessment.

# Cognitive level

'Within-child' factors include affective factors, such as personality type and emotional state, but the aspects discussed here refer to the range of **phonological processing difficulties** which have been identified. The way in which this *causal modelling framework* can be used to portray different theories regarding dyslexia is shown in the BPS (1999) report.

■ **Phonological processing and verbal memory**
The initial problem for young dyslexics turns out to be in identifying the sounds in spoken words – learning to distinguish and manipulate individual phonemes. This function is termed **phonological awareness** and this discovery was a breakthrough in understanding dyslexia. Segmentation and blending skills do develop, of course, and can be improved a great deal through teaching, so methods for detecting weaknesses in older learners need to be more challenging than simple alliteration and rhyme judgement tasks. Therefore, tests are valuable when they require the learner to pick out a phoneme from the middle or end of a word (*phoneme deletion*); transpose phonemes (*spoonerisms*); or time the **speed** at which these tasks are accomplished.

Standardised tests of **segmentation** (rhyming, alliteration, phoneme deletion, spoonerisms – according to age) and **blending** skills are important elements in our armoury of diagnostic tests.

Poor performance in other aspects of **phonological processing** may be revealed through testing and confirm cognitive difficulties underpinning persistent problems with reading and spelling.

Research has shown that deficits in **verbal memory** (the phonological loop of working memory) are almost universal in dyslexia, whilst **visual memory** for symbols is generally unimpaired (see Vellutino et al 1973; Paulesu et al 1996). A model of **working memory** – a system which enables us to hold on to and process incoming information for limited periods of time – was developed by Baddeley and Hitch (1974). Their concept of an **active** central processor with subsidiary loops to supplement the storage capacity of the **central executive** helps us understand memory skills (Figure 2.3). Reduced capacity in the **phonological loop** (phonological processing/verbal rehearsal, etc) would account not only for difficulties with segmentation, but also difficulties in rote learning verbal sequences (times tables, etc), mental arithmetic, remembering messages and so on, so often cited as part and parcel of this syndrome. With normal capacity in the **visuo-spatial scratchpad**, learning strategies which rely on visual and motor memory may be relatively successful.

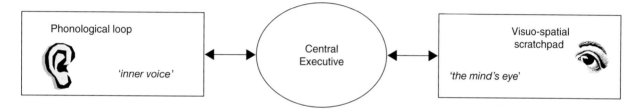

**Figure 2.3** Model of working memory (after Baddeley 1986)

Assessment of auditory short-term memory capacity using a Digit Span test is important from the diagnostic point of view. Of particular interest is the score on **backwards** digit span. This measure is taken as an indicator of **working memory** – the ability to hold items in mind while attending to further demands.

Inefficient/impaired ability to process (store and retrieve) the sounds – but not the meanings of words – leads to other 'symptoms' which can be considered as diagnostic features of dyslexia:

### ■ Vocabulary knowledge
Assessment might reveal restricted acquisition of vocabulary, particularly if compared with higher verbal reasoning. In tests of receptive vocabulary, learners are asked to indicate the meaning of increasingly uncommon single words presented out of context. They are thus forced to access the meaning via the precise sequence of sounds which make up each word. The necessary **phonological representations** may be imprecise, insecure or non-existent.

Such tests differ from verbal reasoning tests. These require an explanation of the *semantic* link between two words (e.g. 'red and blue', which are both *colours*). The words usually relate to everyday concrete items to start with, but gradually become about more abstract concepts (e.g. 'love and hate'). So a higher level of *reasoning* rather than vocabulary is required.

It should be noted that limited reading experience often contributes to lower vocabulary scores in older learners.

### ■ Speech errors
The correct sound (phonological) structure of words whose meanings are known, may not be accurately or completely represented in the mind. This results in mumbled and/or mispronounced (especially multisyllable) words, malapropisms and so forth, as well as words being used incorrectly. Older learners will often report this frustrating tendency and parents/teachers observe it in younger learners.

### ■ Rapid naming
Trouble accessing the *sound* of a word in order to say it, from either its meaning, or indeed its spelling, can result in word-finding problems – that 'tip-of-the-tongue' experience. (This is the reason why many dyslexics find reading **aloud** far harder than reading silently.) Rapid naming tests have become extremely valuable diagnostic tools, since this process is not affected by literacy development. It is thus a measure of a 'pure' phonological skill.

### ■ Fluency
There may be far more difficulty accessing words according to their phonological properties than their semantic similarities. So the speed at which the learner can produce words that start or end with the same sound – e.g. Alliteration and/or Rhyme Fluency compared to words linked by meaning, Semantic Fluency, in the **Phonological Assessment Battery** (PhAB) and **Dyslexia Adult Screening Test** (DAST) – is also of interest.

Research by Wagner et al (see the manual of the **Comprehensive Test of Phonological Processing**) has defined poor performance on measures of **phonological awareness**, **verbal memory** and **rapid naming** as key indicators of dyslexia.

## General ability

As assessors, we would not be doing our job if we did not look beyond dyslexia to see if other cognitive factors were relevant to the presenting problems. Clearly a certain level of cognitive ability is needed for learning, and dyslexic learners of all ages invariably fear that lack of potential is the root cause of their difficulties and need to explore this issue.

Students who appear to have significant emotional or general learning, non-verbal or language processing difficulties, will have a range of special educational needs and referral to other professionals for assessment and advice should be considered – see Chapter 5.

Verbal and non-verbal skills should be assessed. If these are age-appropriate, the potential to cope with the normal curriculum should exist, all other things being equal. (Above-average abilities may be needed in some contexts.)

If both are well below average, general learning difficulties **may** be indicated. If verbal skills (oral communication, vocabulary knowledge, verbal reasoning) are very weak, Specific Language Impairment might be suspected. Problems with visuo-spatial skills as well as general difficulties with problem-solving may contribute to poor performance on matrices tests.

A significant *discrepancy* between verbal and non-verbal abilities (but not necessarily a significant *deficit* in either – see Chapter 11) is of interest in relation to learning styles. The student may find learning 'by doing', by direct experience, very much easier than learning through language – or vice versa. This insight will be valuable to both him and his teachers.

Two points regarding general ability should be made here:

1  Studies have generally shown relatively low correlations (0.4 to 0.6) between IQ test results and exam grades – so we should never underestimate the contribution that good teaching and hard work can make to educational attainment, nor overestimate the significance of IQ scores!

2  Although there is a strong correlation between IQ and reading test scores, the relationship between the two is complex, as discussed elsewhere (BPS 1999; Snowling 2000). Verbal ability, in particular, is considered to be of greater significance for the development of higher-level skills (comprehension and composition) than for mastering the basic coding process, although it is a good compensatory factor at all stages.

# The behavioural level – reading and writing

## Reading

Reading competence should be assessed in three ways and the key issues are **accuracy**, **fluency**, **comprehension**.

■ **Single-word reading**

Performance at this level will not necessarily reveal whether a learner is relying on his sight vocabulary but cannot decode very well. This is where non-word tests are extremely useful – especially if they are timed.

■ **Non-word reading**

Non-words can only be read using phonics. A learner who is inaccurate and/or slow at *decoding* will have trouble working out words which are new for him.

■ **Text reading**

Good practice requires assessment of attainments and strategies when dealing with continuous prose. More than one strategy can be used to access text. Clearly the ability to decode is the secret of success, but whole-word recognition and reading for meaning can supplement and compensate for weak decoding. By carefully analysing how a learner tackles text, through miscue analysis (see page 173) we can identify which strategies are under-utilised and in need of strengthening to promote comprehension.

■ **Timed reading tests**

Enhanced diagnostic power is added if reading tests are timed, since **fluency** of response may still be below par even if **accuracy** and **comprehension** are age-appropriate.

## Writing

Turning now to the **encoding** process, we also need to examine spelling at word and text level and free-writing skills. For older students, in particular, speed of writing becomes an important issue to assess.

■ **Spelling**: for formal purposes, a graded single-word standardised spelling test with a suitable age-range should be used, which will show **accuracy** in relation to the norms for the learner's age.

■ The most useful diagnostic information is to be found, however, by examining spelling in the context of a learner's free writing. Are his word-level skills secure enough to be sustained when attention is focused on composition?

In all cases, however, a careful analysis of spelling errors is crucial and quite often the key to diagnosing dyslexia and working out how to help the learner. Reading may eventually progress since this can be accomplished using more than one strategy; spelling – a task where there is less room for manoeuvre – frequently remains a life-long difficulty. As discussed above, normal development is to 'spell by sound'. Therefore, dysphonetic or frankly bizarre spelling (*sotr* for *story* at 7 years; *kelse* for *careless* at 10 years; *ianzliset* for *anxiety* at 23 years) is of immediate concern and a defining feature of dyslexia.

More often, we see considerable delay in producing fully alphabetic spelling, so phonemes are omitted, or whole syllables (*call* for *called*; *cole* for *could*; *musem* for *museum*; *beging* for *beginning*). It becomes clear in such cases that the sounding-out process is impaired. The process of mapping letters onto speech sounds does not function as it ought, because the learner has difficulty identifying the individual phonemes and remembering them in the correct order. As described earlier, poor phonological awareness and verbal memory are major features of the phonological deficit. It is at this stage of cataloguing spelling errors, that teaching experience – as well as theoretical knowledge – is required. We need to know what 'normal' looks like for a learner, given his age and educational background.

Although phonological encoding skills may be acquired – albeit with considerable difficulty and delay – they rarely become sufficiently automatic to ensure the development of age-appropriate spelling accuracy and fluency at **text level**. Thus the 'knock on' effects of a phonological deficit are apparent throughout life.

- ■ Examining free writing enables us to look at other important variables: handwriting, speed, grammar and punctuation, vocabulary and content – its organisation and structure.

# Environmental influences

## The linguistic environment at home and pre-school

The child who has the opportunity to develop fluent speech and a wide vocabulary when young has a rich and highly specified phonological 'template' in his mind onto which he can start to map letters and spellings. This process continues as he grows older – knowing the meaning of an ever-increasing bank of words and being able to pronounce them clearly makes spelling development, in particular, less problematical. An impoverished linguistic environment makes the whole process of becoming literate that much harder, even in the absence of dyslexia.

If the pupil's first language – and maybe the one he still uses at home and in the playground – is not English, then we need to understand the potential problems beyond the obvious ones stemming from having English as an Additional Language (EAL). His first language may use a significantly different number and range of phonemes; the grammar may be quite different.

## Social and emotional factors

Has the child been to school regularly and with no prolonged absences or changes? Did he adapt easily and has he been settled and happy?

Were there any social or emotional circumstances which adversely affected him during the early years (e.g. death of a parent; family breakdown)? Was teaching consistent and appropriate; learning support adequate and timely?

A child who 'missed the boat' through poor attendance, illness, emotional or behavioural difficulties, poor teaching, etc, during crucial 'learning the code' years can seem dyslexic at 7–8 years old (according to the BPS definition) and certainly needs help. However, he may not have a Specific Learning Difficulty (as per DSM definition) and in such cases, skills can steadily improve once appropriate extra support is put in place.

■ Perusal of school records and reports, and discussions with teaching staff to find out as much as possible about a child's general development in school and learning support put in place, are crucial.

# Specific learning difficulties other than dyslexia

Of course there are other problems with literacy skills which occur – either separately or in conjunction with dyslexia. Poor handwriting is a particular concern.

## Developmental coordination disorder (DCD)/dyspraxia

It is estimated that 10%–15% of the population have handwriting problems (Barnett and Henderson 2004), many associated with DCD. This is characterised by specific difficulties in planning and executing a sequence of voluntary movements (in the absence of any medical reason for the difficulties). DCD may also result in difficulties with speech production, and a range of fine and gross motor skills.

■ The case history will most likely reveal delayed development of motor skills at the pre-school stage – walking, feeding, dressing and self-care. At school, poor fine motor skills – cutting, sticking, drawing, handwriting, fastening clothes and shoes, as well as general 'clumsiness' – and difficulties with PE, changing clothes, ball skills, are often reported. The pupil may be accident-prone and suffer low self-esteem.

■ Learners with DCD are likely to produce poorly formed or illegible handwriting and to complain that writing makes their hand/arm 'tired' or ache. They generally copy and write extremely slowly and have difficulty developing fast, efficient keyboard skills. Layout of written work and maths (execution of diagrams, etc) is probably of a low standard. Poor performance on tests of visual memory, visual-motor integration, manual dexterity, movement and non-verbal reasoning is common.

# Ethical considerations

Fundamental principles underpin ethical practice when gathering personal data and using psychological tests, whatever age of learner you work with. The British Psychological Society's guidelines (see: www.psychtesting.org.uk) provide a sound basis for both organisations and individuals to follow regarding professional conduct when carrying out individual assessments. Key issues are as follows:

- Test users should only work within the limits of their own competence. This means keeping up to date in the subject area. Learners whose presenting problems, or age range, fall outside an assessor's own area of expertise, should be assisted to find an appropriately qualified and experienced professional to help them.

- Competence also means the ability to choose suitable tests in relation to the age and needs of the learner; and to administer, score and interpret the results correctly. Although practical matters such as cost, time taken for administration and scoring are important matters for test users, the fundamental issue here is a sound understanding of basic concepts in educational testing. You need to be able to scan the 'Technical Data' section of any test manual to find essential facts concerning the standardisation sample, the test's reliability and validity, before deciding if it is fit for your purpose. Chapter 11 deals with this topic in some detail.

- Insurance: assessors should be properly insured for both legal expenses and any damages which may be awarded should litigation ensue following an assessment. This protects both parties. (Full members of Patoss are able to join a group policy which provides them with professional indemnity insurance.)

- The purpose and nature of the assessment, how the results will be used and to whom they will be communicated, must be clearly explained to the learner (and/or his parents) and any other professionals involved – beforehand. There **must** be agreement (preferably written) as to who will have access to the results.

- All record sheets and personal data must be stored securely so that only authorised personnel can access this confidential information.

## Summary

Given our knowledge of the normal development of basic skills, the natural history of and diagnostic criteria for particular Specific Learning Difficulties, a sound understanding of educational testing and adequate resources, an assessment will help to understand the aetiology and nature of a learner's difficulties.

Standardised tests supplemented by informal probes focusing on particular skills and knowledge relevant to the learner at that time, together with direct questioning and observation of the learner during the assessment, will all increase our knowledge of which tasks he finds easy and which are effortful and stress-inducing. Our task is to tease out, to the best of our ability, what he can and cannot do: the reasons *why* he is finding particular tasks so difficult, so that learning support can be as effective as possible. The old adage 'teach to the strength whilst remediating the weakness' is always relevant.

The manifestations of a specific learning difficulty will depend on (a) its severity, (b) how it interacts with the pupil's other intellectual and emotional strengths and weaknesses, (c) how effectively – or otherwise – the student has been taught, and (d) how old he is. Therefore, a wide range of individual differences in 'symptoms' exists, as the case studies in this book illustrate. Experience of teaching dyslexic learners and an appreciation of 'the art of the possible' are essential attributes if the recommendations resulting from the assessment are to be useful.

To return to the quotation at the beginning of this chapter: '*Tests don't diagnose, people do.*' The purpose of this chapter has been to provide some of the underpinning knowledge required by the informed and competent assessor, who has a central role in the identification of dyslexia and in effective intervention.

# 3 Practical Aspects of Assessment
## Liz Waine and Sue Kime

'If careful assessment is judged essential for the average school pupil, it is even more crucial in the case of a pupil with specific learning difficulties, whose problems are still frequently misunderstood and are all too often attributed to "laziness" or "lack of ability".'

(Booth 1996)

This chapter considers how the important principles underlying assessment translate into practice. It covers the following:

■ checks to be made before an assessment;

■ gathering background information;

■ selecting appropriate tests;

■ the areas to be covered – underlying ability, reading, writing, phonological skills, memory and other issues;

■ conducting an assessment – assessment plans, location, equipment, rapport, administration, recording and feedback.

# Prior checks

Before starting to plan the session itself, it is important to ensure that an individual assessment is appropriate. Requests for assessment usually come either from teachers, parents, or directly from an older learner. Referrals should only be accepted if there is a legitimate reason for the request, if there has been no other assessment recently, and if all parties involved are willing to collaborate in providing essential information and to discuss the findings. If the referral comes from a parent, has she first discussed matters with the SENCO at her child's school? Most importantly, is the learner himself willing to be assessed? Assuming that all is in order, it is good practice for a written agreement, in the form of an appointment letter, setting out all the terms and conditions, to be signed by both parties.

# Gathering background information

Planning for a full diagnostic assessment should take account of a wide range of background information about the individual's developmental and educational history. Seek details of both pre-school and school experience. Some information that needs to be known before the assessment session can be obtained via questionnaires (see page 183), or a friendly phone call. Much more will be discovered during face-to-face discussions on the day. Questionnaires and interview schedules are useful to ensure that all relevant ground is covered. Many parents will appreciate the chance to reflect carefully before responding to questions about past events. Class teachers/SENCOs need time to collate the information requested. So always give those involved enough time to comply with your request by, say, a week before the assessment.

To make your assessment plan you need to know the main reason(s) for the referral, the learner's date of birth/school year and whether other professionals are already, or have been involved (e.g. speech and language therapists, educational psychologists, specialist teachers). Gather as much documentary evidence as is available – previous reports, school reports and individual education plans (IEPs) before the session – so that appropriate tests and tasks can be prepared. Careful consideration of background information, particularly academic results, together with scrutiny of the learner's work, will facilitate a choice of tests to provide the maximum amount of data in the most efficient way.

## *Information from home/learner*

Parents or carers of primary or secondary pupils are usually the best source of information for details about early development. They will, unless the learner has been fostered or adopted beyond an early age, probably know when milestones such as walking and talking were reached, as well as any family history of learning difficulties. They will understand their child's temperament and interests.

Parents/carers may also be able to provide information about coping strategies and problems not seen at school. In school, the learner may appear well organised. However, this may be because there is a detailed timetable on the kitchen wall noting when each set of textbooks should be taken to school, and mother always packs the sports kit or checks the homework diary! On the other hand, a learner who is apparently well behaved in school may cause problems at home, as the stress and effort of coping all day at school results in tiredness and irritability in the evening.

With older learners, at college or work, such information will have to be gleaned through sensitive questioning. They are not always aware of their early developmental history or may be unwilling to give much information about their background.

Information should also be sought about health, vision and hearing, considering both past and current problems. Check that any vision or hearing aids needed are used during the assessment, where possible.

It is also important to investigate the learner's own priorities for learning, whatever his age. The Code of Practice (DfES 2001) emphasises the importance of involving all children in planning support programmes. Find out about interests and hobbies and, as the pupil moves through secondary school, his curricular needs and aspirations. For an older learner, at college or at work, his career aims, interests, passions and enthusiasms must be included in any intervention plan if it is to be seen as relevant and worthwhile.

## Information from school/college

School/college based information will need to be collated from various sources but the initial enquiry should be addressed to the SENCO/Additional Learning Support (ALS) Manager.

School records are a valuable source of information regarding educational development and academic achievement. Note teachers' comments, for example on performance in relation to effort, as well as reading and spelling test scores, national curriculum tests and other exam results.

In a primary school, the learner's current class teacher will be able to provide information on effort, behaviour, and possibly learning style. In a secondary school or college, it is important to gather information from a range of staff. The art and history teachers, for example, might have very different impressions of the same student.

# Choosing the assessment materials

When deciding which tests to use, ensure best use of the time available by prioritising. Choose age-appropriate standardised tests and prepare relevant, informal, curriculum-based assessments such as phonic checklists or a list of course-related vocabulary. The aim in either case is to gather enough information to provide the starting point for a learning programme that will meet the learner's individual needs. The range of tests used should be broad enough to establish a full profile of the learner's basic skills and strategies, together with evidence of his underlying cognitive skills. Then it is possible to plan appropriate teaching methods building on strengths whilst targeting the development of weaker areas.

It is not the intention of this chapter to prescribe specific tests. Choice of assessment resources will need to take into account the following basic areas but will always depend on the age and stage of the learner. Suggestions for appropriate age-related tests will be considered in Part 2.

# Main areas of investigation

## Underlying ability

As discussed in Chapter 2, an indication of levels of oral language and non-verbal reasoning skills can be useful when planning a support programme. Learners with higher or lower levels of underlying ability may respond differently to certain teaching methods and materials. Furthermore, seriously low results in either or both types of test could indicate the need for referral to an educational psychologist or a speech and language therapist.

In many secondary schools it is common practice to administer non-verbal and verbal ability tests to all students on entry, so it may not be necessary for you to include tests of underlying ability. However, it should be noted that the learner's results on a group **verbal** ability test might be misleading if his literacy difficulties impaired his performance. Individual assessment of his receptive vocabulary and listening comprehension may well be revealing, but you can also make an informal assessment of expressive language ability from his responses and the conversation that takes place during the session. Discussing the content of the learner's free writing is a useful way of identifying any discrepancy between his ability to talk about a subject and to write about it.

## Attainments

### Book knowledge

With a young child, 'book knowledge' should be checked (Clay 2000). Does he know the front and back of a book; the difference between a line and a sentence; the function of a comma? Not all pupils have sufficient knowledge of the *language of literacy* to fully benefit from the teaching they receive.

### Sound-symbol correspondence

Either tactile letters or the whole alphabet printed at random on a single page can be used to assess the young pupil's ability to read and write the names and sounds of single letters. Note his awareness of the difference between vowels and consonants. Use a record sheet to show whether he can confidently give both the *name* and the *sound* of each letter.

With an older student, the extent to which this needs to be assessed will depend on his general level of literacy and so may be decided after reading and spelling have been tested. A learner who, whilst reading a passage of text, shows he can sound out and blend letters to decode unfamiliar words demonstrates his knowledge of letter sounds. Similarly, single-letter encoding skills may be demonstrated through word- or text-level writing activities.

## Reading

It is particularly important when testing reading skills to focus on *how* the learner tackles each task. Knowing that he has a reading age of 8 years and 6 months may facilitate a comparison with peers but will not help in planning a teaching programme. What is needed is information on *how* the learner reads individual words and how well he understands and can make use of what he reads.

All reading tests should be used diagnostically. So, it is very important to record accurately the learner's precise responses using a reliable method of transcription, rather than just using ticks and crosses. Many assessors find it helpful to tape-record the reading and replay it several times when marking-up record sheets. Take careful note of the strategies the learner uses when tackling unfamiliar words. Does he *sound out* all the letters then blend them accurately, or does he attempt to say letter names? Does he attempt to *sound out* irregular words such as *their* but still manage to say them correctly? Does he use this as a diversion strategy while thinking what the word is?

At word level, patterns and rules the learner knows and does not know can be noted and analysed. Can he read words of more than one syllable? Does he differentiate between the vowels and pronounce vowel digraphs correctly? Does he struggle with some consonant blends – and, if so, are these at the beginning, middle or end of words? Do silent letters, 'soft' *c* or *g* confuse him? Does he recognise common letter strings such as *-tion*, *-ight*, and common suffixes: *-ed*, *-ing*, *-ly*?

Bearing in mind the purpose of the assessment, a decision must be made about whether to start with a text-level assessment or a single-word test. If time is limited, assessment at text level will provide the most information about the learner's reading ability in terms of accuracy, comprehension and fluency.

At **word level**, the choice is between an age-appropriate standardised, graded word test and curriculum-based lists. NLS word lists (DFEE 1998) are useful, as well as the vocabulary needed for particular subjects or personal interests. The results of these tests provide valuable information for planning a teaching programme. It may well become clear that a Year 7 learner is still not confident reading words from the NLS list for Reception children and the Key Stage 3 NLS curriculum lists are way too difficult. For an older learner, the emphasis might well be on vocabulary relevant to his course or to his work. An adult working in catering may need to be able to read a range of vocabulary based on menus such as *gateaux* or *spaghetti*. A list of essential subject vocabulary can often be obtained beforehand from the relevant teacher or tutor.

Many phonically-based, structured teaching schemes include graded tests of phonic knowledge at word level. These can be especially useful for younger and weaker readers, as the systematic checking establishes a suitable starting point for instruction.

**Non-word reading** tests give further insights into phonic knowledge and pinpoint decoding skills. They should include both single-syllable and multi-syllable words. A timed test will gauge **fluency**, which is of particular importance with older readers.

**Text-level assessment** yields information not only about the learner's decoding ability but also about his recognition of individual words in context and his comprehension. Standardised tests will give scores for **accuracy, comprehension** and, in some cases, **reading speed**. Alternatively this may be calculated informally using a stopwatch and counting the number of words read within a certain period. It may be helpful to compare a learner's reading speed on fiction and non-fiction curriculum texts. Rate of reading becomes a more important issue during the secondary stage and beyond, when students have to cope with a considerable amount of reading.

The key issue of **comprehension** can only be assessed at text level. The learner might have difficulties here for various reasons. Is he using 'top-down' skills? Is his weak decoding holding him back? Or, are his oral language skills weak? (It is useful at this point to refer to the Gough and Tunmer model: $R = D \times C$ – see page 15.)

To investigate these issues, tests where the pupil reads **aloud** are the most useful diagnostically, since a running record can be made and a **miscue analysis** carried out (see page 173). By categorising the misread words as visually or semantically similar to the target word, as well as looking at how appropriate they are within the sentence or whole passage, it is possible to arrive at a reliable analysis of the learner's strategies. Is he trying hard to read for meaning or is he so focused on decoding that he is not making much sense of what he reads?

A range of texts can also be used to identify independent and instructional levels of reading. An assessor's reading 'kit', therefore, could usefully include passages from reading books, curriculum texts, newspapers or magazines, appropriate for a range of ages and ability levels. Various methods can be used to 'grade' reading materials such as the Fry Readability Graph.

You can download a simple version of this method to use offline from a website (Long 2004).[2]

## Writing

The key issues here are spelling, handwriting, the ability to write and punctuate sentences correctly; and finally text-level skills regarding content, use of language and structure. Of particular interest is the contrast between what a learner will attempt to write independently and his ability to express himself orally. Writing can be assessed via single-word spelling tests, text-level dictation and free writing.

**Single-word spelling** assessment should include a standardised test, possibly supplemented by informal assessment using high-frequency words from NLS lists and relevant subject-specific vocabulary. Spelling should also be examined in the context of free writing and/or dictation. In all cases, note how the learner tackles the spellings – hesitantly, sounding out, or with confidence. Since spelling is nearly always a deep-rooted and persistent problem for dyslexics, this area must be treated sensitively. Learners usually respond positively to a suggestion that they are helping you by 'having a go' at words they are not sure of. This will help your diagnosis.

In analysing spelling it is helpful to consider stages of progression, using the Frith model as suggested in Chapter 2. Remember that children do not suddenly move from one stage to the next; their spelling may show features of more than one stage. Nevertheless, the overall picture of predominant types of error will indicate their level of development in relation to the expected standard for their age.

Look closely for evidence of which specific spelling patterns and rules have been mastered and which are causing problems. For example, is there confusion between vowel sounds? Are the basic consonant digraphs (*sh, ch, th, ng*) known? Do older students know how to tackle multisyllable words or apply suffixing rules? Your analysis will enable you to establish a base line for instruction.

**Handwriting** should also be examined at word and text level to look at the key issues of legibility and fluency, again in relation to age. Significant difficulties with handwriting might trigger investigation of fine motor skills. Again analysis of particular difficulties is vital to plan a programme. Are there individual letters which are difficult to distinguish? Pencil grip is of particular concern in the early years, followed by 'joining up', size, spacing, use of line and so forth (Alston and Taylor 1992). Measurement of rate of writing is complex, as it depends not only on motor skills, but also on fluency of thought and spelling ability. Copying or dictation tasks compared to free writing separate these to some extent.

---

[2]  http://www.psych-ed.org/ – from the home page, scroll down to 'Readability Check'.

Analysis of free writing gives the necessary insights into both **sentence-** and **text-level skills**. Punctuation[3] is closely linked to grammar and needs to be looked at in this light (Pollock and Waller 1994). Content and structure, vocabulary and use of language should be considered at all stages but become increasingly important as learners progress into secondary education. Difficulties with these aspects will nearly always be the focus for learning support at this stage, rather than phonic programmes.

To relieve pressure on the learner during assessment, a sample of **unaided, uncorrected** free writing may be requested from the class teacher in advance. If a school-aged learner is able to provide 'rough' books or examples of 'first draft' writing this will be very useful, but many older learners will be reluctant to provide writing which they know contains errors. It is therefore useful to have stimuli available for use during the assessment session, such as a few sentence starters, *'If I won the lottery . . .'*, or *'Last summer I went . . .'*. If the learner requests support during the writing assessment, make a note of this, perhaps listing spellings provided at the bottom of the page.

## Numeracy

Linguistic difficulties associated with dyslexia can affect the development of numeracy and progress in mathematics in a variety of ways. Visuo-spatial problems can also cause problems in this subject. Neither of these is the same as **dyscalculia** – specific difficulties with number concepts and calculation (Butterworth and Yeo 2004). Dyslexia and dyscalculia should not, therefore, be confused.

Choice of numeracy tests should be based on background information provided when the learner is referred for assessment. Areas to assess may include:

■ counting, both forwards and backwards from a relevant starting point;

■ the ability to read and write numbers and awareness of place value;

■ basic maths appropriate to the age and stage of the learner (e.g. knowledge of the 'four operations', symbols);

■ knowledge of the vocabulary and 'language' of mathematics.

Be ready to use concrete materials where needed – for example, counters and money to explore understanding of basic number concepts. With older learners, fractions are often a sticking point. Here visual representations can help. Can they divide a circle into three or four when asked to show a third or a quarter?

---

[3] For a very accessible short guide to punctuation, see http://www.correctpunctuation.co.uk

# Cognitive processes

## Phonological processing

It is important to remember that assessment tasks for **phonological skills** should not involve processing written words. Assessors should remember that if support is needed this must be in the form of pictures or objects, **not** letters or written words. Phonological awareness should never be confused with phonic skills.

There is a progression in the normal development of phonological awareness and, once formal instruction begins, literacy acquisition and phonological development feed into each other. Therefore age and stage of literacy development will inform your choice of assessment tasks. In order to determine teaching targets, you may need to investigate any or all of the following areas. In addition, fluency or automaticity of skills is an important diagnostic indicator.

### ■ Syllables
If not using standardised tests, you can compile a set of words of varying syllable length to say to the learner. Choose them in advance – you may find it difficult to think of suitable words during the assessment. Remember to include words of only one syllable and present words of different length in random order. Make sure you are assessing the learner's ability to identify how many syllables are in a word and not his understanding of the word *syllable*. For example, with younger learners ask 'How many beats are there in this word – *elephant*?' With older learners you can say 'How many syllables are there in *violin*?' As you ask the question, demonstrate by simultaneously tapping or clapping the syllables whilst saying the word.

### ■ Alliteration and rhyme
The ability to differentiate between the first part of a word and the rest of it is classically assessed using alliteration and rhyme judgement tests. A potential difficulty occurs when the learner cannot remember all the words in the dictated list. To eliminate this possibility, prepare sets of pictures to match the words for younger learners. If segmentation skills at this level are found to be weak they should be addressed in tandem with the teaching of word families using onset and rime schemes.

Tests, however, should always be appropriate to age and stage. For example, it is not necessary to assess alliteration awareness in the learner who demonstrates his ability to read and write the first letter of words correctly.

### ■ Spoonerisms
A spoonerism test is a more demanding investigation of segmentation skills. The additional demands on working memory and blending skills make this an interesting diagnostic tool for the older student, which may reveal intransigent difficulties with identifying and manipulating sounds in words.

With well-compensated adult learners, it may be the one area of phonological difficulty that is identified through assessment.

An informal assessment may be constructed by compiling a list of 10 to 12 pairs of words all starting with consonants or consonant blends. These should be dictated to the learner, who is asked to 'spoonerise' each one. Instructions should be clear, giving an example.

> 'Listen to these two words: *cold day*. Their first sounds are /k/ and /d/. Now say the two words but change over the first **sound** in each word.' Pause to allow the learner a short time to attempt the task, then provide the correct response: *dold cay*. Then give another example for the learner to attempt alone. Point out that the 'new words' are unlikely to be *real* words.

An individual with good segmentation skills will find this task easy and complete each item in about 2 seconds. A high number of errors and/or times in excess of 8 seconds per spoonerism suggest poor phonological processing skills. After the test the assessor should ask the learner how he completed the activity. Did he simply swap the sounds round or did he use visual strategies? Sometimes one will see a learner close his eyes and move his hands as if *seeing* the letters and *moving* them around. This behaviour should be noted.

### ■ Phonemic awareness

Although alliteration requires identification of initial phonemes, further investigation of this crucial skill may still be needed. Deletion of phonemes is a more demanding task and can target middle and end sounds. The learner is asked to repeat words as heard and then again with certain phonemes deleted. For example 'Say *cold*; now say it again but without the /c/'; or 'Say *might* but without the /t/'. The key point to remember as an assessor is to give the instructions using the **sound** of the letter to be deleted, not the name. The pupil who cannot identify phonemes in the middle or at the end of words, or in consonant blends, will have difficulty 'sounding out' words for spelling. These results will therefore be highly informative and helpful with regard to setting teaching targets.

### ■ Rapid naming and fluency

Standardised tests for rapid naming are required in order to compare speeds with age-related norms. You cannot do this informally. Similarly the comparison of alliteration and rhyme fluency with semantic fluency can only be detected through standardised tests. This is an interesting area to explore with an older learner who may be aware of and sensitive about his own word-finding difficulties.

## Verbal memory

When administering a digit span test, make sure that you present the digits at the rate of one per second and take care not to 'chunk' groups of digits. Both forward and reverse span tests should be used. An informal test of short-term memory for random letter sequences may also be useful. Letter spans of increasing length are dictated to the learner in a similar way (but forwards only in this case) and he must write them down. This reflects the skill needed when a learner hears a teacher or tutor spell a word out for him to write down.

Common verbal sequences such as the alphabet, days of the week, months of the year and multiplication tables can be tested informally. Ask younger learners to set out plastic letters in an alphabet arc; older learners might be asked to recite the alphabet or apply this knowledge by using an age-appropriate dictionary, index or telephone directory.

With regard to days and months, although the learner might be able to list the days of the week, can he say which day comes two days before Thursday? Check multiplication tables by asking pupils to recite the full table, not just count on in 2s (2, 4, 6, etc). Many learners with literacy difficulties will be able to do the former task easily but will 'get lost' when reciting the complex sequence of the table, moving from *1 × 2 is 2; 2 × 2 is 4*, to *4 × 2 is 8*, and on to *8 × 2 is 16.*

## Visual and motor processes

It is very difficult to test pure visual memory. The ability to recall and reproduce something seen from memory depends greatly on one's ability to name or label what one has seen. What has been discovered, however, is that some people suffer from visual distortions when reading. It is important to investigate through questioning whether this is the case. If so, referral to an optometrist who specialises in reading problems (and possibly colorimetry) will be an appropriate suggestion. If copying from the board is a problem, one should check that there has been an eye test recently.

Manual dexterity, balance and motor skills are considered in some assessment resources. Decisions about whether to include them will be based on the reason for referral, background information and/or the learner's response to assessment tasks during the session.

# Conducting an assessment

Having decided on the tests you will use, prepare a plan as an aide-memoire for the assessment session. List all the tests you intend to use, allowing space to record observations and noting things you need to remember (e.g. switch tape-recorder on now). Make a note of questions you must remember to ask.

The time needed for an assessment will vary depending on the age and ability of the learner. A young child will not be able to cope with prolonged testing, whereas more time is needed with an older, more advanced learner. Plan rest breaks within the schedule, or consider breaking the assessment up over more than one day.

It is a good idea to mix tests that are likely to be stressful, such as reading and spelling, with other activities probably perceived as less difficult, such as the picture vocabulary test or phonological processing tasks. If using a published battery of tests, it is not always necessary or desirable to use all the subtests.

However carefully the session is planned, you should always be prepared to be flexible. For example, the learner may read at text level better or worse than is expected from the referral information. Have a selection of text passages available. This will ensure that the learner is able to demonstrate the use of context to predict unfamiliar words whilst making enough errors to allow analysis of decoding strategies. Make sure you are familiar with all assessment materials to be used and that all the equipment you need is to hand and ready for use. This may include a stopwatch, tape-recorder, pens and pencils and paper for both you and for the learner.

## *Location*

Arrange for a quiet, undisturbed location. Consider the age and size of the learner and ensure that the chair and table are at an appropriate relative height. Arrange these to make the best use of light sources, but avoid placing him in a position where the sun will glare on the paper.

Most test manuals suggest that the assessor should sit at right angles to the learner. This allows her to observe the learner as he completes each activity. It is useful to have some sort of 'barrier' to stop the learner seeing test record papers and the notes made during the session. This could be an open file or book cover. If you are right-handed sit on the right-hand side of the learner. You can then hold up the file cover with your left hand whilst recording test notes with the right. If you are left-handed the opposite will apply.

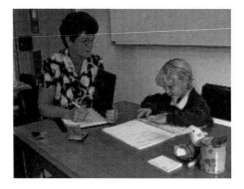

**Figure 3.1** Right-handed assessor

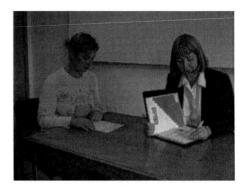

**Figure 3.2** Left-handed assessor

# Rapport

It is important to make sure that the learner is settled and relaxed from the start. He needs to know the purpose of the assessment and what is likely to happen; how long it will take, and that he can have a comfort break whenever he needs to. Allow time to get to know him, to ask about his favourite activities and lessons/subjects, what he finds difficult and what he would like to be better at.

There is a fine distinction between being a *teacher* and a *tester*. As a teacher or tutor we all want to ensure that our learners are successful and that they do not fail on any activities we give them. However, the purpose of the assessment is to determine not only what the learner can do, but also the point at which he begins to fail. We need him to find some activities difficult and make errors so that we can analyse them and identify the strategies he is using. The progressive difficulty of tests should be explained and the learner prepared for 'failure' at some point. For example, with a primary child, one could say: *'I use this test with much older students so it will get difficult. I don't expect you to get it all right so you must not feel bad when it gets too hard.'* With older learners, explain the need to see where the difficulties lie in order to plan a support programme.

Throughout the assessment give appropriate praise and encouragement. However, you should avoid giving feedback as to whether responses were right or wrong. Try to respond with a neutral phrase such as 'thank you' or 'OK'. Most learners will be aware that a test is becoming more difficult, but are more likely to keep trying if they are not given feedback that confirms an error. Praise and encouragement at the end of each activity enables you to be supportive and maintains good rapport with the learner.

# Administering tests

Good preparation will enable you to move smoothly between activities, noting if the learner appears to need a break.

When administering standardised tests it is vital to follow the instructions in the manual. This will give full details of the procedures and will usually tell you exactly what to say. Each test is standardised using these procedures, so deviating from them will invalidate your results. If necessary you can explain to the learner that you are following a script.

Deciding on cut-off points can be difficult, particularly in reading or spelling tests if a learner becomes distressed by his 'failures'. It is quite legitimate in these circumstances to discontinue testing before the test's stated cut-off point is reached. If this is the case, a standardised score cannot be calculated and this should be made clear in the report.

# Recording

It is vital to keep a written record of the learner's responses to all activities. *How* an activity was tackled is as important as *how well* in both standardised tests and informal tasks. You should not rely on memory but make notes throughout. Tell the learner *'I need to make notes to help me remember what you have done when I write my report.'*

Observe closely and note the way the learner tackles each task. How confident does he appear? Does he make eye contact with you? Does he sit straight on his chair? Does he carefully consider all options before responding or appear to make impulsive guesses? Does he close his eyes when asked to recall information, suggesting he might be visualising detail or alternatively that he needs to 'cut out' all other distractions? What does he do when a test becomes difficult? Does he become noticeably tense or restless? The assessor should take note of all these aspects of behaviour and relate them to all the other relevant information.

# Feedback and discussion

A well-planned assessment will identify a learner's strengths and weaknesses in a time-effective way. It will reveal underlying difficulties and also provide the specific information needed to plan an intervention programme. At the end of the session you will be able to discuss how the assessment went, making a point of stressing any areas of competence that were noted. Ask the learner how he now feels and acknowledge his co-operation during the session. Most learners, or their parents, will want to know what your main impressions are straight away. You should therefore be prepared to deal with this, being honest about what is immediately obvious, but explaining that you now need time to analyse all the results carefully and think things through. It might be possible at this juncture to discuss options regarding learning support. Explain when the report will be available and what opportunity will be available to discuss its implications.

## Summary

- Before beginning an assessment it is important to know the reason for referral and to gather a range of background information.
- Referral and background information is necessary in order to choose appropriate assessment procedures, which will include formal, standardised tests and informal assessment methods.
- Written records must be kept of the learner's responses in each assessment activity and of his reactions during the session.
- The aim of the assessment is to gather enough information about the learner's cognitive abilities and literacy skills to identify areas of strength and difficulty, in order to plan an intervention programme.
- Treat the learner as an active and equal partner during the assessment session as well as in subsequent discussions about the results and their implications for the future.

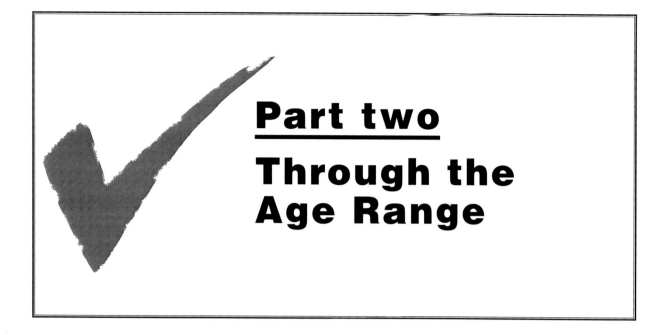

# Part two

# Through the Age Range

# 4 The Foundation Stage

Prue Ruback

'It is not intended that children should be sat down and assessed and tested in any formal way.'

(Pascal, in QCA 2003)

The recent *Foundation Stage Profile* (FSP) (QCA 2003) heralded a new observational approach to assessment. It built on the stepping-stones and early learning goals from the *Curriculum Guidance for the Foundation Stage* (QCA 2000) and promoted well-planned, practitioner observations, over time, for children in the Foundation Stage.

The FSP replaces statutory baseline assessment and is therefore the starting point for early years practitioners. However, it is not intended as a screening tool for dyslexia and so does not go far enough in providing the detailed information which might help a primary teacher or SENCO to identify potential dyslexics or in assessing what additional help might be needed.

A major concern for early years practitioners is in knowing which of children's observable behaviours are developmental and which signal potential specific learning difficulties. All children develop at their own unique rate and comparisons between individual children are not helpful in determining which children might be at risk for dyslexia.

Careful observation by early years teachers provides assessment information to SENCOs, to help determine whether individual children have needs which warrant additional resources and/or support. This information, accumulated over time, can be supplemented by parents, nursery staff, other early years practitioners and by the children themselves.

Early years practitioners will already be alert to children who do not conform to the usual expectations for the Foundation Stage. This initial concern would go beyond children who are just shy and disinclined to say much, or those children who are unable to cut with scissors, or catch a ball. Home circumstances and environmental factors differ widely and for many young children simply starting nursery or reception can be a daunting experience.

However, it is useful to consider 'early-indicators' which might warrant further investigation, or referral for specialised assessment.

In the Foundation Stage, 'at risk' children might demonstrate problems with:

■ oral communication: speech, language and vocabulary;

■ phonological awareness;

■ alphabet knowledge;

■ short-term (working) memory skills;

■ attention and perseverance on tasks.

Related factors might include:

■ family history;

■ book knowledge;

■ other physical factors.

# Assembling a family history

For new entrants to the reception class it is important to gather as much information as possible from the child's family, where practicable.

Any family history of literacy difficulties could be significant. There is much accumulated evidence that where a child has a dyslexic parent there is an increased likelihood of that child being at risk for dyslexia (for a review, see Lundberg and Hoien in Fawcett 2001).

Early years practitioners need to be very sensitive here: some parents are unwilling to reveal their own literacy problems to a teacher, sometimes they simply do not know the real cause of their literacy difficulties, or attribute literacy acquisition problems to other causes, like interrupted schooling, ill health, or truancy.

Sometimes dyslexia skips a generation, so a grandparent, or other family member might have dyslexic difficulties. This information, if proffered, can be very helpful in assembling a full case history.

**Action:** note down . . .

■ any references to family literacy difficulties, which although in isolation may not seem relevant, will help to build up a picture of a dyslexic profile;

■ information on siblings/family members who had problems acquiring literacy skills.

# Communication skills: speech, language and vocabulary

 *Oral language ability is an essential precursor of written language development.* 

(Wood, Wright and Stackhouse 2000)

An increasing proportion of children begin school with poor speech and language skills. This phenomenon is quite separate from those children for whom English is an additional language. Having English as an additional language is not a special need in itself. However, if parents report scant, indistinct or poor speech in their home language, this is a cause for concern and advice should be sought from a bilingual speech and language therapist.

Foundation Stage children with poor spoken language skills are at risk for literacy difficulties (Stackhouse and Wells 2001). They are more likely to have problems acquiring the literacy skills they need in Key Stage 1 and beyond, so all aspects of language need to be carefully monitored and examples noted.

Within the context of the Foundation Stage Profile, practitioners will already be monitoring how children initiate conversation, use language to interact with other children, use talk to imagine, sequence, modify and explain actions and to negotiate with others. These complex language skills enable children to clarify their thinking and are an essential part of their social, emotional and cognitive development.

Early years teachers should have some understanding of language acquisition, so that they know the normal pattern of language development and can pinpoint significant deviations from the norm.

The average 5 year old should be able to:

- repeat a sentence of twelve syllables, e.g. *'I'm going to play in the park with my granddad'*;

- give four objects in order: *'Bring me your coat, scarf, hat and Wellingtons'*;

- understand *what*, *where*, *who*, *when* and *why* questions;

- use a sentence of more than five words in length.

A helpful screening test, from which these examples are adapted, can be found in Gross (2002).

**Action:** note down . . .

- family information concerning lateness to speak;

- references to non- family members finding it hard to understand the child;

- references to the child being later than others in attaching names to everyday objects or colours;

- examples of substituted 'near miss' words – e.g. *lamp post* for *lampshade; water pot* for *watering can.*

- examples of persistent jumbled phrases and spoonerisms like *beddy tear* for *teddy bear* and *par cark* for *car park;*

- bizarre forms of words, such as *suebegi* for *spaghetti*, *plisters* for *slippers*, where the listener cannot identify the correct target word.

## *Vocabulary*

The average 3 year old has a vocabulary of over 1000 words, which rapidly increases, so that a 5 year old should have an active vocabulary of over 3000 words and a passive vocabulary of substantially more. The Foundation Stage Profile states that a child at the end of the Foundation Stage should show 'control of a range of appropriate vocabulary'.

The difficult question for early years practitioners is to know what constitutes *appropriate* vocabulary. Some children who fall within the dyslexic continuum have enormous difficulties with word-finding and this could be apparent even within the Foundation Stage.

Early years practitioners will be aware of children who take inordinately long to communicate their meaning and who use gesture to accompany their speech output. So when engaging in outdoor sand play, searching for the target word *spade*, the child might ask for the *digging thingy*, accompanying this with digging movements. It is not that the word *spade* is outside their vocabulary or experience, but that they cannot retrieve it when they need it.

Early years teachers might notice children who frequently have their hands up during circle time or 'show and tell', but have forgotten what they want to say when invited to respond.

Taken individually these factors might not seem significant but together they can contribute to the dyslexic profile.

The National Literacy and Numeracy Strategies place emphasis on quick, pacy, interactive oral work, but the very activities designed to engage children may mask the dyslexic who cannot respond and retrieve the correct answer in the time available.

**Action:** note down children who . . .

- have word-finding difficulties;
- have their hands up but cannot answer appropriately;
- attach the incorrect verbal labels to everyday items;
- use gesture, pointing or mime to convey meaning, more than other children do.

# Phonological skills

In the Foundation Stage children should show '*an awareness of rhyme and alliteration*' (QCA 2003).

Since the seminal work of Bryant and Bradley (1985) there has been a growing acceptance of the crucial link between phonological skills and learning to read and spell.

**Phonological awareness** means the ability to distinguish sounds within words which are heard, not written; aural not visual.

**Alliteration** means identifying the first sound (*onset*) in the word: the *J* in *Jack*. **Rhyme** relates to the last chunk of the word (the *rime*): the *-ack* in *Jack*. By 5 years most children will be able to supply alliterative examples, e.g. giving other children's names beginning with *J* → *Jill, Jenny, Jamal, Jo*.

Games which require children to make judgements on the basis of 'odd man out' – where three out of four objects begin with the same initial sound; 'pencil, pin, *scissors*, paintbrush' – will help teachers to identify children with poor phonological skills.

Foundation stage children should be able to recite nursery rhymes and to join in with them, supplying the missing rhymes, thus '*Jack and Jill went up the . . . .*'

According to Stackhouse and Wells (1997), normal 5 year olds should be able to give one rhyming word for a given target, so children could be asked to supply various words (and non-words) to rhyme with *spot* → hot/got/cot/lot/mot/dot/rot/what/not.

Intact phonological skills allow children to read and spell words *by analogy* (Goswami and Bryant 1990). Phonological impairment is a strong indicator that a child might be at risk for dyslexia, so any training or enrichment activities that help children to develop their phonological skills will be of benefit. In the NLS *Lunchbox* video materials, reception teachers can be seen modelling rhyme activities to give children practice in supplying suitable rhyming words:

> *Humpty Dumpty sat on a chair*
> *Looked around and saw a . . . . . . (bear/pear/fair/hare)*

Appropriate activities can also be found in the *Progression in Phonics* (PIPS) materials and in the *Early Literacy Support* (ELS) materials.

However, early years practitioners should be aware that rhyme training alone has not been shown to generalise to segmentation at the phonemic level, so training in phoneme awareness and phoneme deletion (what is *slip* without the *s*? → lip) will be crucial for children who are exhibiting problems in this area. (For further discussion see Muter 2003.)

Foundation stage practitioners might also consult Layton et al (1997) for activities and games which help to develop phonological awareness.

**Action:** note down . . .

■ any child who is unable to recite a nursery rhyme;

■ any child who is unable to identify the odd man out in sequences like cat/*pig*/bat/mat;

■ any child who is unable to generate rhymes: cat/fat/mat/ ? . . . (hat, sat, pat);

■ any child who is unable to classify words or objects on the basis of the first phoneme (alliteration);

■ any child who is consistently off-target when playing I-Spy, because they have not understood that it is the first phoneme which is required to guess the target word.

# Alphabet knowledge

Research has shown that secure alphabet knowledge is the single, strongest predictor of later reading proficiency. Children in the Foundation Stage should be able to '*link sounds to letters, naming and sounding letters of the alphabet*' (QCA 2003).

By the end of the reception year, children should demonstrate 'knowledge of grapheme/phoneme correspondence' (NLS) and be able to use this knowledge to read and spell simple words.

Early years practitioners have a vast repertoire of activities to teach grapheme/phoneme correspondence, including sound tables, sound of the week, and practising letter formation and identification. Teachers should be alert to children who, despite the specific and structured phonic teaching advocated by the DfES in the NLS, PIPS and ELS materials, cannot associate graphemes with their correct phonemes and who cannot reliably identify both upper- and lower-case letters, by the end of the reception year.

**Action:** note down children who, by the end of reception . . .

■ cannot write their own full name correctly;

■ cannot correctly identify 26 lower-case letters of the alphabet;

■ have difficulty identifying the 26 upper-case letters;

■ cannot sequence the alphabet orally and with plastic letters.

# Short-term (working) memory

It is hard for class teachers to reliably assess the speed and efficacy of working memory in very young children. Practitioners should be alert for children who have more difficulty than their peers in following a set of oral instructions. As a general rule, 4 year olds should be able to recall three numbers or items in the correct sequence and 5 year olds should be able to repeat back a sentence of at least twelve syllables.

Three areas of the FSP deal with memory skills:

■ **Communication, language and literacy**
  • Language for communication and thinking: point 7 – using talk to sequence ideas;

  • Reading: point 7 – retells narrative in correct sequence.

■ **Mathematical development**
  • numbers as labels and for counting: point 6 – counts reliably up to ten everyday objects;

  • point 7 – orders numbers up to 10.

■ **Creative development**
  • point 4 – sings simple songs from memory;

  • point 6 – recognises repeated sounds and sound patterns and matches movements to music.

Across the Foundation Stage, practitioners should note the child who suddenly forgets what to do next, when children are following a set of procedures to make a model or bake some biscuits. Such children can be also observed in PE, dance and drama as being several seconds behind peers in their responses, often because they are watching other children, to see what to do next, since they cannot remember/interpret the teacher's oral instructions.

**Action:** note down children who . . .

 have difficulty using numbers as labels;

 cannot repeat a four-item sequence or set of actions;

 cannot retell a simple story they have just heard;

 fail to remember class jingles, routines and chants;

 have great difficulty in sequencing a set of three picture cards in correct order;

 are unable to play 'my aunt went to market and bought . . . .'

# Attention and perseverance

Children in the Foundation Stage should be able to sustain concentration and remain on task for a period of time.

The FSP *Personal, social and emotional development*: dispositions and attitudes, point 8, states 'maintains attention and concentrates'.

Practitioners will be alert to children who cannot concentrate during story time, who wander from one activity to another without any sustained engagement and who become overly frustrated or anxious when they cannot derive immediate success. These children find it difficult to complete tasks because of limitations to short-term, working memory and possible language processing problems. Such children may also shun literacy-based activities, in favour of construction toys or free-play situations.

Johnson, Peer and Lee (2001) describe an experiment where they noted reception-age children who consistently avoided reading-type activities. These children were later found to have literacy difficulties at age seven.

**Action:** note children who . . .

 are unable to sustain concentration (e.g. during story time);

 fail to persevere with table activities, so do not complete the task;

 seem to wander from one activity area to another, with minimal engagement;

 find it hard to play collaboratively (e.g. in the role play area or with outside equipment);

 consistently avoid reading and writing activities.

# Conclusions

Within the Foundation Stage setting it is difficult to form any definitive conclusions about children who might have specific learning difficulties. One risk factor alone does not constitute a dyslexic profile. Some children grow out of their problems, and there could be a host of other causal factors, such as *otitis media* (glue-ear), which might have delayed some aspects of cognitive development, or family/environmental/social/emotional factors.

It must also be remembered that some children within the Foundation Stage who exhibit *none* of the risk factors discussed above, will later go on to be assessed as falling within the dyslexic continuum. Such children may begin school with no apparent difficulties or mask them very successfully. Their specific problems with literacy only manifest themselves at the end of Key Stage 1, when the constraints and content of the National Curriculum make too many demands on them.

**Actions:**

■ observe closely;

■ record carefully;

■ have the confidence to realise when the problems noted require the involvement of other professionals, such as the special educational needs coordinator, speech and language therapist, the educational psychologist, the child's key worker, or a specialist teacher.

Johnson, Peer and Lee (2001) concede that '*observing young children at play, then appears to be an effective method of monitoring children who might be "at risk".*'

The quotation at the beginning of this chapter – '*It is not intended that children should be sat down and assessed and tested in any formal way*' – appears in the introduction to the FSP training materials (QCA 2003), written by Professor Christine Pascal. It is an approach which makes good sense for very young children in the Foundation Stage.

Well-informed practitioners hold the key to the early identification of children who might be at risk for dyslexia: continuous assessment and observation will provide the background evidence needed for subsequent intervention.

# 5 Primary Level
## Margaret Bevan and Val Hammond

'A stitch in time saves nine.'

(early 18th century saying)

In this chapter we shall look at:

■ particular considerations for the primary school age range from 5 to 11;
■ children who learn differently;
■ assessment at the primary level
  1 background information
  2 underlying ability
  3 attainment – reading, writing, spelling, maths
  4 cognitive processes;
■ outcomes of assessment;
■ modes of intervention and referral to other professionals.

# Particular considerations for this age range

By the end of Key Stage 1, children may have fallen at the first hurdle of learning to read and write. However, it is at this stage when it is possible to make the most difference by appropriate interventions. As children approach transfer to secondary schooling, effective support can help prevent increasing difficulty and distress caused by poor literacy skills and ineffective learning strategies.

We have seen in the previous chapter how information gathered in the Foundation Stage can identify the 'at risk' child. This monitoring process will continue at Key Stages 1 and 2, but will now include careful monitoring of progress in literacy and numeracy. The information gathered through national curriculum tests (NCTs, formerly SATs) and through groupings for intervention programmes such as ELS, ALS, FLS[4] will be important.

---

[4] ELS: Early Literacy Strategy; ALS: Additional Literacy Strategy; FLS: Further Literacy Strategy.

A huge learning curve takes place during the primary stage of education. This is a time of fast development, keeping pace with ever-increasing demands. By the time a child leaves primary school he is expected to have mastered functional and fluent literacy skills. Children who have not reached this stage face the daunting prospect of entering secondary school, knowing that they are already falling behind their peers. These children often learn in a different way, and through an individual assessment it is possible to identify the additional support they need.

# Children who learn differently

**David** (age 6 years 10 months)
David is struggling to develop more than a basic sight vocabulary, but uses context well in reading. He has found it hard to learn his individual letter sounds and is reluctant to write more than one sentence. His mother reports that he was slow learning to speak. When he did, his speech was full of mispronunciations, especially with polysyllabic words. This difficulty is still obvious as he struggles to say *capital letters* and *consonants*, which he pronounces as *catipal* letters and *consternants*. Any suggestion that he has general language difficulties is belied by his good comprehension and verbosity. But when he tells his news, his speech is circumlocutory and full of 'whatchammacallits' as he struggles to express himself clearly and access the words he needs. Sometimes the names he uses demonstrate a clear image being accessed rather than a verbal label: for example, he talks about a *camera-picture* rather than a photograph; a *flat* egg rather than a fried one. His mother reports that he found nursery rhymes difficult to remember, although if they were sung he could recall them more efficiently. She also noted that he was poor at carrying out instructions. If told to go upstairs, put on his pyjamas and clean his teeth, he would remember to do one only. Yet he appears to be much better than his friends at building Lego models and is a keen little footballer. She is very concerned, as his father, a highly successful engineer, was only identified as dyslexic when he went to university.

**Joanna** (age 9 years 7 months)
Joanna is reluctant to write. She is unhappy about her handwriting, which is large and untidy. Her pencil grip is awkward – she uses four fingers rather than the traditional tripod grip. She produces far less written work then her peers, although she has excellent ideas for stories and a good wide vocabulary when speaking. She likes reading and enjoys drama. She finds it hard to structure her writing, which tends to be disorganised. She sticks with 'safe to spell' words, yet still makes careless spelling mistakes.

Joanna also experiences difficulties with maths: she has problems with place value (beyond three digits). She still does not know her tables and rarely contributes in mental maths sessions. Her untidiness and poor layout add to her difficulties with written work.

School staff acknowledge these difficulties, as well as her general tendency to be untidy and fidgety. They concede that she may not be reaching her potential, but do not see a major problem. Her parents, however, are most anxious about the fact that Joanna is unhappy at school and hates games and PE.

Learners like David and Joanna are noticeable in class as being different from other children; they are also very different from each other. Specific learning difficulties have many guises. Some children will identify themselves very early as they struggle to learn alphabet sounds. Others will cope with the early stages of reading through developing a good sight vocabulary, but may never manage to crack the alphabetic code completely. Children with milder problems may not be noticed until a later stage, when their difficulties with spelling and writing at an age-appropriate standard become apparent.

# Assessment

The major issue in assessment should always be what can be done to help these children with their difficulties whilst utilising their strengths. This is what makes assessment more useful than screening. Screening has its place in identifying those who might benefit from an in-depth assessment.

# Background information and observation: what would one notice/look for at this age range?

Parents' concerns should always be heeded. In the first few years of education they are very accessible as they take and fetch children from school. They are the people who know their children best and become worried if they do not make the same progress as peers or older siblings.

Children themselves are only too aware of others who are racing ahead with reading. Anxiety frequently accompanies difficulties at school and can show itself in unwillingness to get ready in the morning, tummy aches and 'clamming up' about the school day.

The classroom teacher will be aware of the child who is not learning as expected. In primary school, children are predominantly allocated one class teacher. She has often had experience of hundreds of children passing through this stage of education, so is a hugely important source of information. The classroom assistant works closely with individual children and may have a useful contribution to make from her perspective.

Children's ability to attend and concentrate in class or at home is a useful developmental pointer. Are they constantly fidgeting? Is it hard to get them to respond? The development of spoken language is always a key area to observe. Are they expressing themselves easily and fluently or are there immaturities or difficulties in articulation (e.g. *lellow* instead of *yellow*) or in use of language (e.g. *Miss telled me*)? There may be a tendency to interpret words (e.g. '*Pull up your socks, all of you*') at a literal level!

Informal questioning of children themselves during the assessment should add even more to this growing picture. Do they like reading? What do they read? Do they enjoy writing? What do they enjoy most at school? What do they think they are good at? What, if anything, do they dislike? What would they like more help with? The ensuing conversation can be very illuminating and will tell much about the pupil's self-esteem and how their difficulties have been managed in the school setting. Nothing is more pleasurable than to hear a pupil with very weak reading skills say he loves reading and books. This will be a pupil who has been handled sensitively, who has been asked to read books that were manageable, who has been involved in the pleasure that books can give by being read to and by paired/shared reading (Topping 1995).

# Underlying ability

For this age group it is important to look at underlying ability using tests that are appropriate for age and stage. Tests need to cover both verbal and non-verbal skills:

| | |
|---|---|
| **British Picture Vocabulary Scale (BPVS)**<br>• 3 years–15 years 8 months | Measures receptive vocabulary – that is, the words that a learner understands. A useful test, interesting and non-threatening – throughout Key Stages 1 and 2, it can illuminate how much the pupil might understand of what goes on in the classroom. |
| **Non-Reading Intelligence Tests 1–3 (NRIT)**<br>• 6 years 4 months–13 years 11 months | Administered orally to a group, so do not disadvantage the child who cannot read well. |
| **Raven's Coloured Progressive Matrices (RCPM)**<br>• 5–11 years | Tests non-verbal reasoning and is appropriate for the very young. |
| **Raven's Standard Progressive Matrices (RSPM)**<br>• 6 years to adult | Usually more appropriate than RCPM at Key Stage 2 and above. |

Interpreting these test results is a key issue. A noticeable imbalance between verbal and non-verbal scores can indicate specific learning difficulties affecting verbal or, alternatively, non-verbal skills, if either is below average (i.e. below a standardised score of 85). The profile of a dyslexic child may well show significant or comparative deficits in verbal skills. If he has a relative strength in non-verbal reasoning, his teachers and parents will need to know that he finds it much easier to learn in a practical way, rather than purely by listening and talking.

Weak vocabulary underpins many pupils' difficulties with reading and comprehension. For those with significant deficits in vocabulary acquisition, referral to a speech and language therapist might be appropriate. In the school context, it is always wise to recommend vocabulary extension. Above all, access to books and reading material on a regular basis should be recommended. Listening to stories on tape containing good-quality prose helps to develop vocabulary, especially if an adult discusses the content with the child.

# Reading attainments

**Reading** should be assessed for skills in decoding, for knowledge of sight vocabulary, for comprehension and fluency at text level.

A good place to begin formal assessment is with a **single-word reading test** to provide an indication of starting level: this will be helpful when looking at the other aspects of reading:

| | |
|---|---|
| **Wide Range Achievement Test 3 (WRAT–3)**<br>• 5–75 years | Both appropriate for this age group. |
| **Graded Word Reading Test**<br>• 6–14 years | |
| **Word Recognition and Phonic Skills (WRaPS)**<br>• 4 years 6 months–9 years | Requires the reader to point to the correct word from a choice of five, when a stimulus word is given orally. Two scores are provided, which show the child's success with regular compared to irregular words – a helpful diagnostic tool. This can be used as a class or individual test and is very easy to use and score. Useful when the pupil is very young or very weak. |

**Nonword reading tests** can quickly identify the pupil with limited decoding skills:

| | |
|---|---|
| **Nonword Reading Test**<br>• 6–16+ years | Has the advantage of being timed, so that accuracy and fluency are assessed. |
| **Phonological Assessment Battery (PhAB)**<br>• 6–14 years | There is a nonword reading subtest within this, but it is not timed. |

If these are not available, it is possible to devise an informal probe from your own lists of non-words using phonic patterns drawn from the NLS lists for the appropriate Key Stage.

Tests of **reading in context** provide vital information about the child's ability to use picture and context cues.

| | |
|---|---|
| **Individual Reading Analysis**<br>• 5 years 6 months–11 years 2 months | Both are widely used and generate age-equivalent scores for accuracy and comprehension. |
| **New Reading Analysis**<br>• 7 years 5 months–13 years | |

| Diagnostic Reading Analysis • 7–16 years | Measures accuracy, comprehension and speed; provides a useful comparison with listening comprehension. |
| --- | --- |
| Neale Analysis of Reading Ability (NARA), second revised British edition • 6 years–12 years 11 months | Differs from the above in that you can help the child with words they cannot read.[5] |

Comparing reading accuracy and reading comprehension can be illuminating. Generally one would expect them to correlate. It is therefore significant when there is a discrepancy between the two.

This may well be so for dyslexic learners who may read inaccurately because they miss out function words (such as *the, a, for, of*), yet do obtain good scores for comprehension. Sometimes they will be unable to say a word, yet know what it means; or they may mumble over words they find hard to pronounce. All this will affect their accuracy score, yet they do gain the sense of the passage.

Similarly it is significant when the score for comprehension is lower than the one for accuracy. This may be due to a 'barking at print' approach where the effort to decode prevents meaning being fully accessed, or it may mean that the child has more generalised language comprehension difficulties. In this case it can be useful to re-run the test using a parallel set of test passages purely as a listening comprehension activity, or else to use the **Diagnostic Reading Analysis** referred to above.

It is important to observe the strategies used in reading. Is the child a logographic reader, relying mainly on the shape and appearance of words? How far does he have knowledge of alphabetic principles (see Chapter 2)? Does he recognise initial letters but guess medial and final sounds? In what ways does he approach text? Does he take cues from context or pictures? Does he self-correct? Miscue analysis will provide additional quantified evidence of reading strategies (see page 173). Sometimes signs of visual discomfort are obvious when the child frequently loses his place or rubs his eyes.

### ■ Recommendations

The general principles of intervention in reading at this stage are to develop word-, sentence- and text-level skills.

It is important to target text-level skills by encouraging the enjoyment of reading – developing fluency, vocabulary and comprehension. It is to this end

---

[5] However, this raises the question of whether the scores obtained for comprehension really reflect independent reading ability.

that approaches such as paired reading, repeated reading and listening to stories can be recommended.

Books for independent reading should be at the correct level, i.e. where the child can achieve 95% accuracy, with a high interest factor. There should be opportunities for repeated reading as, for example, in play reading, and (for Key Stage 1) rhymes and familiar tales. The beginning reader needs to map speech to print; for weak readers, paired or repeated reading can be a useful strategy to achieve this. Tape-recording his own reading will allow him to map his own speech patterns to printed words as he reads along with the tape.

Helping the pupil to 'interact' with a text rather than just reading it, may prove helpful from the earliest stages. This means visualising the content, thinking about it, forming an opinion, reading between the lines and discussing the content with another person.

At word level it is impossible to separate reading and spelling interventions, as they are interrelated and draw on each other. The use of multisensory techniques, which involve all the senses, will build up spelling skills, which will then feed into reading accuracy.

Automatic recognition of **key words** is an essential part of reading fluency in the early years, but these words are often irregular and carry little meaning out of context. Furthermore they are not easily pictured. It is important to explain in your report that such words need to be embedded in sentences to enable the child to recall them. Games are essential here for *over*learning.

Drill cards using key words in context are useful – for example:

| | |
|---|---|
| **Come** | **Can I come and play?** |
| *front* | *back* |

The word is placed on the front of the card and a simple sentence (created by the child) on the back. The sentence on the back embeds the word in real language and can be flipped over as a memory trigger for the child if he does not immediately recognise it in isolation.

## Sound-symbol correspondence

Testing **sound-symbol correspondence** may well be necessary at this age range. It should not be taken for granted that it has been fully mastered. This can be assessed using tactile letters in the early stages and should include the consonant digraphs *ch, th, sh, ng*, as well as single letter sounds. Confusion between letter names and sounds is a cause of common spelling errors such as *rm* for *arm*.

| Checking Individual Progression in Phonics (ChiPPs) <br> • 6–7 years | Requires the reading of a graded series of real and non-words which clearly identify the stage of breakdown of **phonic knowledge**. It provides follow-up work with the provision of the relevant unknown word families. |
| --- | --- |

### ■ Recommendations

Multisensory methods and personal picture cues will help to alleviate confusion between vowel sounds. Encouraging mastery of pure sounds and drawing attention to the way they are pronounced will help children distinguish between pairs of voiced/unvoiced consonants such as *b/p, d/t, v/f/, z/s*.

The teaching of phonics is an integral part of spelling tuition. Many young dyslexic pupils will find isolated phonemes difficult to recall, so vowel digraphs and diphthongs can be taught within rime chunks. However, specific attention to phonemes can be addressed through a wealth of published programmes. In your report, emphasise the importance of multisensory strategies which encourage the use of hearing, seeing, saying and writing letters, alongside the use of movable letters.

## Writing attainments

Any analysis of **spelling** skills should consider the pupil's performance in a single-word spelling test and a piece of free writing.

### Single-word spelling tests

All single-word spelling tests give a spelling age and can be used diagnostically. Each has its own advantages.

| Helen Arkell Word Spelling Test <br> • 5–17+ years | Has a short-cut route to the point of breakdown which means that there is less need to exhaust the pupil before reaching the level of errors from which one learns the most. Also contains follow-up suggestions. |
| --- | --- |
| Parallel Spelling Tests <br> • 6–15 years | Admirably suited to whole-class testing, this single-word spelling test has useful follow-up suggestions. <br><br> Rising steeply in terms of difficulty, it permits regular re-tests as it has several parallel sets of spellings. |
| WRAT–3 Spelling Test <br> • 5–75 years | Has two parallel forms and covers a wide age range. |

As in reading, you can make useful judgements about a pupil's level of writing vocabulary by analysing which year group's key vocabulary he has mastered. Lists of Key Words for dictation can be taken from the National Literacy Strategy.

It is also essential to look at spelling in a piece of unaided free writing to see whether the spelling in context is as accurate as single-word spelling. This gives an idea of how automated spelling patterns are. Lack of automatic spelling skills is often illustrated by failure to use written vocabulary which matches levels of spoken English. The pupil may tend to stick to 'safe' vocabulary.

Analyse spelling development using Frith's stages (see Chapter 2). A child who is not spelling by sound (i.e. alphabetically) may attempt to spell words by remembering how they look. The word *jumped* might be written as *jmudpe*. (The 'e' is often added as he realises the word does not look long enough!) There is no attempt to follow the order of speech sounds.

As the child moves into the alphabetic stage his phonic knowledge is matched by his segmentation skills. There may be a development through *jpt, jupt,* and ultimately *jumpt,* as more speech sounds are identified. Alphabetic spelling of high-frequency irregular words such as *sed/said, wos/was* herald this stage, and should be seen in a positive light initially.

Correct spelling of a word such as *jumped* indicates that the child understands the significance of the past tense marker -*ed* and is attaining competence at the **orthographic level**.

Children may by now be reading irregular words fluently but not yet spelling them correctly. The process of refining spelling, noticing double and silent letters and so on, is easier for the pupil with the 'inner voice' as he reads. This voice is continually matching speech sounds to the representation on paper and becomes tuned to pick up irregularities (e.g. I don't hear the /b/ at the end of *thumb*).

When looking diagnostically at **spelling skills and strategies** note the **level** of phonic knowledge revealed: single letters, blends, digraphs, common letter strings (e.g. -*tion*). Are there sounds in words for which the child has no phonic representation? For example, does he write *lok* instead of *look* (oo), *bening* instead of *burning* (ur), *crach* instead of *crash* (sh).

Are errors phonetic, semi-phonetic or sometimes bizarre (e.g. *kerm* rather than *garden*)? Does the child vocalise whilst sounding out spellings or is he quick and confident? Are common irregular words spelled correctly or are the correct letters present but in the wrong order? Is he displaying knowledge of spelling rules?

### ■ Recommendations

Before discussing methods of addressing spelling difficulties it is vital to consider the pupil's level of phonological awareness (see below) since this underpins the ability to spell 'logically' (Frith's alphabetic stage). If the pupil has phonological difficulties and is introduced to a structured spelling scheme, he is likely to pay attention to the visual similarities in the lists of words, but not relate them to the sounds. This should be emphasised in your report. Phonological skills and spelling need to be addressed *together*.

Good readers and spellers use analogy as one of the sub-skills for attacking unknown words. They decode these words by linking the visual patterns or sound patterns of words they already know to the unfamiliar word. Thus if they know *rain* they can read *train, explain, complain*, etc.

A spelling programme based on rhyme analogy can help the child to develop and use this skill. Recommend the teaching of word families containing the same sound patterns. A larger chunk is easier to recall than single phonemes blended together. For example: *oil* rather than *oi*, *eat* rather than *ea*.

It is important to combine this work with auditory work that involves **saying the sounds**. (Wood, Wright and Stackhouse 2000). Cumulative and structured dictations for rehearsal will test the effectiveness of the teaching.

There are a number of tried and tested schemes that work at phoneme level. These schemes will need additional work on phonemic awareness. Research (Muter 2003) indicates that this level is crucial; rhyme training alone does not generalise to segmentation at the phonemic level.

For the spelling of **irregular words**, advise the use of other strategies such as mnemonics, simultaneous oral spelling, colour coding of difficult parts of words, or visualisation. Focus on spelling errors found in the child's free writing, as these are words he will want to use most often.

## Free writing

The root cause of difficulty with free writing may be spelling, handwriting, grammar, organisation, or memory difficulties.

To judge writing **speed**, older pupils, who are able to write more extensively, can be asked to mark the text at five-minute intervals. In the book *Assessing and Promoting Writing Skills* (Alston 1995) there are standardised norms for writing speeds in Key Stage 2, alongside some excellent guidance for writing analysis.

The free-writing sample should be considered in terms of 'secretarial' or technical skills and content. These areas can be further subdivided: secretarial into spelling, handwriting, grammar, presentation and punctuation; content into creativity, style and structure.

When looking at **handwriting**, consider handedness, letter formation/ proportion, style (cursive/print/mixed) pencil grip/control and paper position. It is important to be familiar with the handwriting policy of the school. Look for difficulties with letter/number orientation, particularly *b/d, p/q, 9/p* or the use of capitalised versions of *B* and *D*. This is more significant after the age of seven, as these behaviours are common in the younger child.

Consider whether grammar and punctuation are age-appropriate. These are inter-related. It is clearly unrealistic to expect understanding of the possessive apostrophe or of clauses at Key Stage 1. On the other hand, there is sometimes refreshing evidence of style and creativity in the work of a child whose writing and spelling are almost undecipherable. Do not forget to look out for and acknowledge this almost buried talent – it needs to be nurtured and encouraged.

### ■ Recommendations

In looking at handwriting, analyse the main cause of a pupil's problems. A checklist (e.g. Taylor 1999) is useful for involving the learner in identifying and targeting his own particular difficulties. Recommendations could include some fine motor exercises, postural or pencil grip changes.

Storyboards could help with the visual presentation of a sequence of ideas. These can later be written up with either words, sentences or paragraphs under each picture – a useful differentiation task for classroom teachers who want to address all ages and stages of ability in writing. Writing frames, like storyboards, help to structure ideas, cut down the writing load and help towards an understanding of sentence structure. Mind maps can be used to plan writing; tapes used to record thoughts prior to writing. Word processing can support extended pieces of writing where drafting and redrafting is required.

## *Mathematics*

The **Graded Arithmetic-Mathematics Test** (age range 5–12 years) gives a standardised score and 'mathematics age'. It can be administered in 30 minutes and gives an assessment of overall mathematical attainment, but can also be used diagnostically. For weak readers there is the option to administer it orally.

Does the child understand how to count a number of things? Does he count on his fingers? Does he confuse the words 16 and 60, or reverse numbers when he writes them down? Does he have a clear number line in his mind and can he see number patterns? Does he show signs of poor working or rote memory skills? What strategies are used for calculating? Does he confuse operational signs? Are there basic concepts he has not grasped? Can he estimate? Does he misinterpret maths language? Are there difficulties with layout and recording? Is he impulsive or considered in making responses?

Remember to look at maths performance together with visual integration and handwriting in order to identify any visual perceptual and spatial awareness difficulties.

### ■ Recommendations

Your main recommendation for this age group will be the use of concrete materials such as Cuisenaire rods, counters, Diennes blocks, bead or paper abacus and games to reinforce concepts and mathematical language. Many pupils will have difficulty with accurate counting, sequencing and directional problems. Using physical activities, visual imagery and stories linked to real-life situations can help a child talk through a particular problem or understand a concept. Money can be a useful mediating route. Concepts need to be fully understood at a concrete level before they are abstracted into symbolic representations.

Number patterns need to be pointed out: '*I know that 2 plus 5 is 7; therefore 22 plus 5 is 27.*' Avoiding the teens can help at this stage, as the 'teen' decade, especially the words *eleven* and *twelve* often prove to be a stumbling block in this generalisation process.

Squared paper helps with the organisation and accuracy of calculations. Advise that children are encouraged to jot down as they calculate; draw word problems; use colour to code signs or place value of numbers. Special care is needed with maths language. This needs to be considered as any foreign language: one needs to be able to work from maths language to symbols and vice versa. The latter will require the child to make up maths stories from a presented equation. As work progresses it is useful for them to create an individualised maths reference book containing a glossary of vocabulary and 'worked' examples with written explanations.

## *Cognitive processes*

### Phonological processing

The main standardised tests for this stage are:

| Pre-School and Primary Inventory of Phonological Awareness (PIPA)<br>• 3 years–6 years 11 months | Assesses letter knowledge and phonological awareness at syllable, onset-rime and phoneme level. |
|---|---|
| Phonological Abilities Test (PAT)<br>• 5–7 years | Contains four phonological awareness tests (two rhyming and two segmentation tasks), a speech rate subtest and a letter knowledge subtest. |
| Phonological Awareness Battery (PhAB)<br>• 6–14 years | A battery of eight phonological tests and one semantic fluency test that can be used as a measure against which to compare his phonological fluency. Appropriate throughout Key Stages 1 and 2. |

| Comprehensive Test of Phonological Processing (CToPP) <br> • 5 years–24 years 11 months | Measures phonological awareness, phonological memory and rapid naming (so useful in defining a range of difficulties). Much faster to administer than the PhAB, but is American; transferring words into an English form takes some practice. |
|---|---|
| Sound Linkage <br> • 7 years to adult | Contains an excellent diagnostic test which finds the breakdown points in development of the ability to segment words. Begins by testing at syllable level, then rhyme, then phoneme. Follows up with suggested work at the weakest level before moving on to the next stage. |

In assessing phonological skills, consider how fast is the child's response. Does he sound out/blend syllables? Does he make use of rhyme? Can he manipulate phonemes? Does he need pictures to aid memory? Does he exhibit word-finding difficulties? Is there a contrast between phonological and semantic fluency? The dyslexic with weak phonological skills may well achieve an average or better score in semantic fluency, while the pupil with general language difficulties, or English as a second language, will find accessing words by meaning as difficult as accessing them by sound. One also needs to notice the naming difficulties of some pupils, who – in all tests – will be slow in accessing words they need.

### ■ Recommendations
As stressed above, phonological skills underpin the ability to spell and in turn to decode. Support for this function should focus on the level at which the pupil is experiencing difficulties. This could be with syllables, rhymes or phonemes. Work on phonological awareness must be done through auditory (not written) work, but should always be linked in with spelling work.

## Memory

Testing Digit Span is the traditional way of identifying strengths and weaknesses in verbal memory. Working memory (see page 21) is a skill required for word blending, for mental arithmetic, for following instructions and explanations. Both forward and reverse tests require efficient use of the 'inner voice'. This can be dependent on efficient phonological skills. Look at the Dyslexia Institute website (www.dyslexia-inst.org.uk) for a Digit Span test which can be used at this age range.

Informally, it will also be necessary to find out whether a child can remember the days of the week, months, alphabet sequence, times tables, date of birth, address and telephone number. This analysis will highlight difficulties to be addressed in an individual teaching programme or through class work.

Note how quick responses are and the strategies used – for example, visualisation, vocalisation, 'chunking' of digits.

### ■ Recommendations

Memory is a difficult area to train in isolation and it is better to recommend that strategies be applied to specific tasks. Explain that it is helpful to link one modality to another to enhance memory. For instance, when copying from the board, read aloud what is being copied. Recommend also strategies such as colour coding, visualisation, mind mapping, mnemonics and acronyms (Bristow, Cowley and Daines 1999; Saunders and White 2002).

Memory is inextricably linked to attention and listening. Encourage the use of strategies to aid listening: maintaining eye contact, thinking about what is being said and visualising the content. Strategies for the teacher may be to call the child by name before giving instructions, give instructions in small steps, and ask the child to repeat what he has been asked to do.

To remember common sequences, recommend use of movable letters for alphabet sequencing games. Advise that days of the week and months of the year are not taught at the same time. Days can be taught one by one and colour coded to the child's particular interest for each day.

## Personal organisation

Organisational skills may be informally investigated through observation and questioning. The child might have difficulties with keeping personal possessions in order, getting started on activities, following the school timetable, or finding his way around school.

### ■ Recommendations

Strategies for resolving these practical difficulties, which often cause a disproportionate amount of anxiety and irritation, should be suggested, working in partnership with parents and school staff.

## Visual skills

Does the child skip or repeat lines when reading or omit words? Does he use his finger to point or complain of print moving? Does he have difficulty with near- or far-point copying, rest his head on the desk whilst writing or reading, or occlude one eye? Does he suffer from excessive fatigue or show signs of squinting or repetitive blinking? Is his presentation of written work 'all over the place', perhaps with writing moving away from the margin? Does he have difficulties catching a ball?

Visual problems may be optical (eye behaviour, scotopic sensitivity) or cognitive (e.g. perception and memory). Sometimes a child might have a weakness in visual perception – his mind does not make sufficient sense of what his eyes see. The **Beery Buktenica Visual Motor Integration Test** (VMI) has two subtests assessing visual perception and motor skill. Many pupils learn to use the mediating route of language to talk through what they need to analyse visually, so it is important to note the strategies used in this test as well as the Raven's. Difficulties with visual perception might contribute to problems in reading, drawing and aspects of maths involving spatial skills.

### ■ Recommendations

Optical problems may lead to referral to an optometrist specialising in reading difficulties and/or use of coloured overlays. Advice about where the child sits in class, enlargement of worksheets, large print books, computer fonts and screen colour might be appropriate. Templates for guiding layout in maths, letters, written work can be very helpful.

## Motor skills

| Motor Screening Test<br>• 7 years to adult | Ten tasks which inform the tester of what difficulties to look out for; follows up with excellent activities for structured programmes of work. |
| --- | --- |
| Movement Assessment Battery for Children Checklist<br>• 6–9+ years | A classroom screening and monitoring assessment which provides normative data of movement and manual dexterity. |
| Beery Buktenica Visual Motor Integration Test (VMI)<br>• 2–18 years | The 5th edition has excellent sections which look in great detail at the stages of normal motor development in the very young child. |

It is important to note: poor coordination affecting sport and activities such as bike riding; bad posture; untidiness in the classroom; slow and/or untidy writing; awkward pencil grip.

### ■ Recommendations

Popular physical activities – swimming, trampolining, dancing – can be helpful. Both Portwood (1996) and Johnson Levine (1991) contain useful programmes and advice.

# Outcomes of assessment

Just as detectives link the evidence gleaned from a crime scene, you too can link the evidence from test results and behaviour to form conclusions about the nature of the child's difficulties. Let us now look at the way test results were used to draw conclusions about the problems that David and Joanna, introduced earlier this chapter, were experiencing (see Figures 5.1 and 5.2).

> By emphasising each child's very sound attainments, acknowledging and specifying their difficulties and suggesting ways of addressing them, the children themselves, their parents and teachers were provided with the information they needed to make constructive and relevant Individual Education Plans.

# Modes of intervention

Having identified your pupil's strengths and weaknesses from assessment, and formulated your conclusions, the next step is to address the difficulties through a programme of teaching support. This can be done on several levels that take into account the waves of intervention recommended in the Code of Practice, individual support, group support and differentiation within the classroom.

An individual support session can be specifically tailored towards a child's individual needs and small achievable targets set. These can be laid out in a cumulative and sequential programme of lessons delivered by a specialist teacher. Alternatively advice may be given to enhance group work the child may already be receiving through the ELS, ALS and FLS programmes already in place. A more general level of advice should be given to the class teacher to aid in the differentiation of class work.

## When to refer to other professionals

Assessment profiles for some children can be very complex and we must know when it is appropriate to refer on to other professionals in the field. It is important to obtain the right advice and help at this stage. The table on page 76 is useful for reference.

**David** (age 6 years 7 months)

| Standard Deviation | −3 | −2 | −1   0   +1 | +2 | +3 |
|---|---|---|---|---|---|
| Test | Well Below | Below average | ← *Average* → *range* | Above average | Well Above |
| Vocabulary – BPVS | | | | X | |
| Non-verbal – Raven's CPM | | | X | | |
| **Reading** – NFER Graded Words | | X | | | |
| Non-words – PhAB | | X | | | |
| **Spelling** – Young's Parallel | | | X | | |
| Verbal memory – Digit Span | | X | | | |
| **PhAB:** Alliteration | | | X | | |
| Rhyme | | X | | | |
| Spoonerisms | | X | | | |
| Fluency – alliteration | | X | | | |
| Fluency – rhyme | | X | | | |
| Fluency – semantic | | | X | | |
| Rapid naming – pictures | X | | | | |
| Rapid naming – digits | | | X | | |

David's high-average scores in the BPVS and the **Ravens Coloured Progressive Matrices** contrasted sharply with his lower scores in literacy attainment. Five (six, including non-words) below-average scores were noted in his performance on the **Phonological Assessment Battery**, providing clear evidence of underlying phonological processing difficulties. There were also indications of limited auditory short-term/working memory capacity. The assessment findings support the opinions of David's parents and his teacher that he is a boy of high average ability who may have inherited a family trait for specific learning difficulties. Indeed, he presents with what is sometimes regarded as a 'classic' dyslexic profile.

The suggested programme included combining oral rhyming games with a structured spelling programme, working at the onset and rime level to start with. The need to use multi-sensory methods and to work on one regular pattern at a time, with just two or three high-frequency irregular words, was emphasised. David's parents were taught Paired Reading techniques and agreed to read with him every day using this method.

Figure 5.1

**Joanna** (age 9 years)

| Standard Deviation | −3 | −2 | −1 | 0 | +1 | +2 | +3 |
|---|---|---|---|---|---|---|---|
| Test | Well Below | Below average | ← *Average* → *range* | | | Above average | Well Above |
| Vocabulary – BPVS | | | | | X | | |
| Non-verbal – Raven's CPM | | | X | | | | |
| **Reading** – NFER Graded Words | | | | X | | | |
| Non-words – PhAB | | | | X | | | |
| Comprehension – NARA | | | | | X | | |
| **Spelling** – Young's Parallel | | | X | | | | |
| Verbal memory – Digit Span | | X | | | | | |
| **PhAB** – all subtests | | | | X | | | |
| Visual-motor – VMI | | X | | | | | |

Joanna presented a very different picture. Her case history revealed a host of mild difficulties with fine motor skills since infancy – using cutlery, dressing, cutting and sticking and so on. Seen in this developmental perspective, her awkward pencil grip and untidy handwriting suggested specific difficulties with motor coordination. This diagnosis was supported by her weak performance on the VMI for motor skills. Joanna's vocabulary, PhAB scores and word-level reading and reading comprehension were all comfortably within the average/high-average range for her age. Her spelling was fully alphabetic (e.g. *booles* for *bullies*) but weaker than her reading. It was suggested that the 'careless' mistakes she often made when writing (e.g. *qwik* for *quick*) stemmed in part from not having established secure motor patterns for common words.

An analysis of her handwriting showed that size of midzone letters, height of ascenders, and letters not sitting on the line were the chief problems. A programme to address these issues one at a time was suggested. Plans to develop her touch-typing skills and increase her use of the computer were also made. It was agreed that the quantity of written work expected from her in class and for homework would be reduced. The use of simple writing frames was recommended. Her writing speed would be monitored with a view to perhaps applying for extra time during her Key Stage 2 tests.

The implications of reduced verbal memory capacity when trying to follow instructions and explanations or do mental arithmetic were explained. Strategies to reduce these problems were recommended to Joanna and her teacher.

Figure 5.2

The following table is useful for reference:

| Other professionals | Referral for: |
|---|---|
| **Educational Psychologist** | • assessment of cognitive ability<br>• need for statutory assessment<br>• emotional/behavioural issues<br>• child and family guidance issues |
| **Speech and Language Therapist** | • unclear speech; problems with articulation – stuttering, stammering, etc<br>• language development – delay or disorder<br>• social communication difficulties |
| **Paediatrician\*** | • possible developmental delay<br>• possible medical conditions<br>• possible autistic spectrum disorder |
| **Paediatric Physiotherapist or Occupational Therapist\*** | • concerns regarding motor coordination difficulties/clumsiness |
| **Optometrist/Orthoptist\*** | • concerns regarding visual acuity/comfort/perception, squint, etc |
| **Audiologist\*** | • concerns regarding hearing |

\* A referral from the school doctor or GP is usually required before a consultation with these medical professionals.

## Summary

- If children are experiencing difficulties in literacy acquisition, this is the stage when it is possible to make most difference by appropriate intervention.
- Children with dyslexia and/or other specific learning difficulties often learn in a different way.
- The purpose of an individual assessment is to identify the additional support they need.
- Use age-appropriate tests to investigate underlying ability, attainment, and cognitive processes.
- Look for clusters of difficulties which make up an individual pattern.
- Decide on the most appropriate modes of intervention and consider when to refer to other professionals.

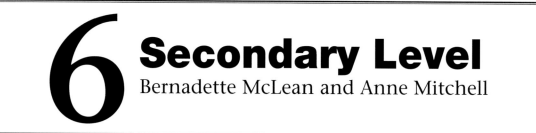

# 6 Secondary Level
## Bernadette McLean and Anne Mitchell

'Who would expose workers to an organisation which required them to work for ten different bosses in one week, in three or four different work groups, to have no work station or desk of their own but to be always on the move? What sensible organization would forbid its workers to ask their colleagues for help, would expect them to carry all relevant facts in their heads, would require them to work in 35-minute spells and then move to a different site, would work them in groups of thirty or over and prohibit any social interaction except at official break time? The typical secondary school . . . .'

(Handy 2000)

# Particular considerations for pupils in secondary education

It is unsurprising that the transition to secondary school can be challenging for many pupils, not just those with specific learning difficulties. Less severely dyslexic pupils may not have been suspected as having specific difficulties until this stage, when there are many new challenges to contend with:

- more teachers and a complicated timetable (some schools operate on 6-day or 8-day timetables) needing different equipment on different days;

- more and new subjects, with an increasing amount of subject-specific vocabulary; as well as words which have different meanings in different settings (e.g. *scale, set, bug, file*);

- more reading and writing demands in most subjects, and more homework;

- more demands for rote learning (e.g. foreign vocabulary, formulae).

The whole nature of education becomes more fragmented at this stage. It becomes harder to capture a full picture of the learner when so many teachers are involved. Class teachers at secondary level may be ill equipped to deal with pupils with low reading skills. Their training has skilled them to teach their specialist subjects, but not even teachers of English will have been trained to teach the early stages of reading and writing.

# Indicators of difficulties

Whilst the difficulties seen during the primary school years (see Chapter 5) may well persist into the secondary years, this may not be the case if there has been effective intervention. What may not be obvious is that literacy skills apparently mastered have not reached the stage of being automatic, so that tasks are often more effortful for the dyslexic pupil than for his non-dyslexic peers. Moreover, after secondary transfer, new difficulties and problems arise because of the changing environment and increased curricular demands.

After GCSE, pupils may specialise and focus on a narrow range of subjects. Prior to this, however, they are expected to be 'generalist', rather than specialist, and to achieve right across the curriculum. A tendency to do better at practical subjects where less reading and writing is involved is often noticed at this stage.

Particular areas of concern to consider at this level include:

■ inaccurate reading (e.g. misreading examination questions);

■ slow reading; losing the thread of longer texts, poor skimming and scanning skills and trouble getting the main idea;

■ difficulties in acquiring subject-specific vocabulary; understanding, reading and spelling technical words;

■ the demands of studying a foreign language, in particular French;

■ ineffective note-taking skills from books or in lessons (listening and writing at the same time): problems in planning, organising and structuring written work;

■ use of restricted vocabulary that is easier to spell, thus masking the true level of understanding and expression;

■ legibility and speed of handwriting; punctuation and presentation;

■ difficulties in proof-reading own work: spotting errors;

■ personal organisation: having the right equipment and materials in the right place, at the right time; time-keeping and meeting deadlines;

■ tiring more easily than peers – more prone to examination stress;

■ low self-esteem, possibly leading to behaviour problems and truancy.

# Purpose of assessment

At this level, parents, pupils and their teachers are increasingly aware of the significance of externally marked examinations and will ask for an assessment to determine the need for examination access arrangements (JCQ 2004), such as extra time. There is a greater interest in doing well at GCSE and A-level than at Key Stage 3 national curriculum tests, because GCSE results are qualifications which greatly influence what happens afterwards. Success in achieving places in further and higher education and in employment can depend on these results.

All specialist teachers carrying out assessments, which might be used for examination arrangements, should hold a qualification recognised by the Joint Council for Qualifications. (A list of these 'approved' qualifications is published annually and updated throughout the year on their website: www.jcq.org.uk.) Further guidance for specialist teachers, school and college staff on this topic is available in the Patoss/JCQ guide (Backhouse, Dolman and Read 2004). Independent practitioners should be aware that the JCQ regulations require collaboration between Centre staff and the specialist teacher or educational psychologist carrying out assessments for this purpose.

# Gathering background information

As emphasised throughout this book, collecting background information about a learner is important prior to an assessment. At secondary level, where the student has a number of teachers, and his parents are less likely to come into school, the easiest way of gathering this information is through the use of questionnaires or checklists (see page 183). Responses should enable the assessor to identify at-risk factors associated with dyslexia, such as family history and late speech development, and to highlight any indicators of dyslexia, such as delay in learning to read. Reviewing the information from subject teachers may reveal not only recurring strengths and weaknesses but also inconsistencies between performances in different subjects. In addition, other barriers to learning as well as previous learning support may be documented. All these factors must be considered when analysing assessment results and drawing conclusions.

Subject teachers will provide invaluable information about how well an individual copes in different environments, where there are different protocols and expectations. Every effort should be made to interview them, or at the very least the Year Tutor. A phone call to discuss the learner will greatly improve the quality of the information you obtain and help to foster the co-operative approach needed with this dynamic process. It will also provide opportunities for further questions.

The student himself, is, of course, a primary source of information at this stage. He is generally able to explain where his strengths and weaknesses lie; what he has found helpful or frustrating; and above all his current aims, ambitions and particular concerns.

Let us now introduce two students: Abdul, in Year 7, whose parents have asked for an assessment, and Susie, in Year 10, referred by her SENCO.

> **Abdul** is twelve years old and is having ongoing difficulty in mathematics. All developmental milestones were reached at an appropriate age. Abdul enjoys school, particularly sports and technology, but finds maths difficult and English 'boring'. His recent school cognitive ability scores were all within average bands; but he is in a low set for maths and has not received any support. He is a normally happy and well-adjusted boy who wants to be an engineer.

> **Susie** is fifteen years old and is studying for her GCSEs. She has always struggled with reading and spelling and there is a family history of spelling difficulties. There were no problems with her early development, though her medical history shows that she suffers from migraines and is asthmatic. Although shy, she is popular in school and gets on well with peers and adults. Normally well-adjusted, she is becoming anxious and her confidence is reported to be fragile.
>
> She lacks fluency and speed when reading; she uses her fingers to track her place and she does not comprehend easily. She tends to spell phonetically, but this strategy does not always work with longer words. She frequently finds it hard to understand what is being asked of her.

We will consider these students again later in this chapter.

# Planning the assessment session and choosing materials

The purpose of the assessment will usually determine the most appropriate tests, and influence the choice of standardised or criterion referenced tests.

In practice, both are likely to be used (Chapter 3 deals with these issues in greater depth). In the examples given above, however, it will clearly be important to use formal tests for Susie, since the assessment results may well be used as evidence of need for access arrangements in examinations. For both students, informal probing of specific difficulties with certain subjects or study skills will be needed in order to plan a programme of support.

When choosing tests for secondary-aged students, it is particularly important to ensure that the test age-ranges are appropriate: some well-known tests have their 'ceiling' at around 13 years of age. It is equally important to observe and investigate the strategies used by students while engaged in responding (Levine 1994). With all tests you can ask learners how they arrived at the answers when they have finished, without invalidating the results.

Observation during the assessment can provide useful diagnostic information and insight into the amount of time and effort expended on tasks. 'Compensated' learners (a term used to describe dyslexic learners who have managed to develop age-appropriate basic skills) use a range of strategies to cope with literacy and numeracy tasks in the classroom. Learners may, for example, sub-vocalise in order to remember information, or use a pointer (pen, finger) to keep their place when reading. Such information can be used as supporting evidence when describing individual strengths and weaknesses. The assessor can also use the information to help formulate a teaching programme which utilises the strategies already used, or to recommend developing alternative ones.

It should be noted here, that, in our experience, learners who are far behind may well still demonstrate difficulties in areas inappropriate for this age range, such as basic phonics, common sequences, times tables and so on. A good principle when testing pupils with dyslexia is 'never assume anything'. So be prepared, but do use care, tact and diplomacy to make assessment relevant for those who are 11 years and older. Young people at this stage often have fragile self-esteem. 'Image is everything.'

In the hands of a skilled assessor, a well-planned session will not only yield test scores but a wealth of diagnostic information about the pupil.

## *Underlying ability*

'Intelligence tests do not come close to assessing all the developmental functions needed to succeed at school' (Levine 1994). Nevertheless, tests of general ability offer pointers to how well pupils will cope with aspects of the curriculum. Furthermore, the tests suggested below are particularly appropriate for dyslexics, as they do not involve reading or writing, unlike many of the group ability tests commonly used in schools. The downside is that most of them have to be administered individually.

| British Picture Vocabulary Scale (BPVS), 2nd edition<br>• individual administration<br>• 3 years–15 years 8 months | A measure of receptive vocabulary (the vocabulary that is understood but not necessarily used); often a good predictor of potential academic achievement. Takes about 10 minutes.<br><br>Supplementary norms for pupils with English as an additional language (EAL) are available. |
|---|---|
| Raven's Standard Progressive Matrices (SPM)<br>• individual or group<br>• 6 years to adult | A test of non-verbal reasoning where visual observation, ability to see the pattern or shape, and logical thought are required.<br><br>Useful for evaluating potential in students with poor language skills or those with EAL. |
| Naglieri Nonverbal Ability Test (NNAT – Multilevel form)<br>• individual or group<br>• 5–17 years | Also uses progressive matrices to assess general problem-solving ability in a way that is unbiased for those with language difficulties. Takes 20–25 mins. |
| Wide Range Intelligence Test (WRIT)<br>• individual administration<br>• 4–84 years | An American intelligence test that specialist teachers can use.[6] Four subtests measure verbal and visual abilities, and the scores can be aggregated to give a general ability measure. Takes up to 45 mins. |

For a dyslexic pupil, the **BPVS** can reveal abilities not apparent in the classroom if his expressive vocabulary is affected by poor word retrieval, or if he is unwilling to join in class discussions for other reasons. A good score can be encouraging and bode well for the student's ability to deal in the currency of learning – i.e. spoken language in the classroom. A poor score, however, should be treated with caution, particularly with older pupils, since it may be a consequence of poor reading abilities. Poor readers often avoid reading; however, reading feeds into vocabulary acquisition increasingly as pupils grow up. The language of books is not the language used with peers. A pupil may seem to have good expressive skills in communicating with his friends, but this may not indicate an extensive vocabulary. One solution is to provide vocabulary enrichment by listening to books on tape or CD.

The student's expressive language abilities can be considered during the course of conversation and when listening to his responses to reading comprehension questions. His teachers will also be able to tell you about his ability to express himself orally. His free writing may give you an indication of his quality of language – even if it is badly spelled!

---

[6] Unlike the WISC (for children), WAIS (ages 16–89), and WASI (ages 16–89), which are closed tests and therefore only available to psychologists to administer.

If the **Raven's Standard Progressive Matrices** is used as a group test, one loses the opportunity to look at strategies used by the student when tackling the problems. Does he use verbal strategies to solve problems or does he obtain the answers very quickly, suggesting a more visual, holistic approach?

The **Wide Range Intelligence Test (WRIT)** has a high correlation with Wechsler IQ scales and the norms were developed on the same population as the **WRAT–3**. Administration is straightforward and if time is short, the subtests could be administered in separate sessions.

# Attainments

## Reading

### ■ Word-level tests

Single-word reading tests tap decoding skills and sight-word knowledge without the clues of context and grammar. Persistent difficulties with these aspects of reading are in keeping with the BPS definition of dyslexia (see page 17). Testing can be informal, using words from the National Literacy Strategy or subject-specific words, or formal, through standardised single-word reading tests.

| | |
|---|---|
| **Graded Word Reading Test**<br>• 6–14 years | Two parallel versions for re-testing; untimed. |
| **Wide Range Achievement Test 3 (WRAT–3):** *Reading*<br>• 5–75 years | Two parallel forms of graded words; untimed (also contains spelling and arithmetic tests). |
| **Test of Word Reading Efficiency (TOWRE)**<br>• 6 years–24 years 11 months | Two subtests – Sight Word Efficiency and Phonemic Decoding Efficiency. Results are combined to give an overall score. |
| **Nonword Reading Test**<br>• 6–16 years | Two parallel forms; also timed; provides error analysis columns on record sheet to help identify phonic patterns the student does not know and needs to learn. |
| **Wordchains**<br>• individual or group<br>• 7 years–adult | A timed test (about 10 mins) of letter and word recognition. |

It is also a good idea at this stage to have an idea of how *automatically* (i.e. quickly) the pupil can recognise words.

❝ *It is well established that difficulties in automatic word recognition significantly affect a reader's ability to effectively comprehend. . . . Many readers who struggle to learn to read are able, with appropriate instruction, to compensate for initial reading problems by becoming accurate decoders, but fail to reach a level of sufficient fluency to become fast and efficient readers.* ❞
(Hook and Jones 2002)

The **Test of Word Reading Efficiency (TOWRE)** measures this aspect of reading, as it compares both real-word and non-word reading under timed conditions. A discrepancy between the two subtest scores is particularly revealing. Dyslexics are often far worse at the non-word subtest because of their weak decoding skills.

The **Two-Minute Reading** test (of real words) in the **Dyslexia Screening Test** can be used for the same purpose.

**Wordchains** can be administered to a group and therefore used for screening, or individually as part of the diagnostic procedure.

It should be noted that word recognition does not make the same demands as reading words aloud, nor is it possible to observe errors and strategies.

### ■ Oral prose-reading tests

Prose-reading tests, read aloud, measure comprehension, but disadvantage readers whose efforts to decode leave little energy for understanding. Note whether the student has to re-read the passage in order to answer comprehension questions, or can respond straight away; and whether he puts the answers in his own words or quotes verbatim from the text.

Assessors are advised to explore comprehension difficulties and check whether the problem is language-based or due to a reading difficulty. This can be done informally by using a passage from one of the parallel forms of the prose reading tests to read to the pupil, or for him to read silently, before asking him comprehension questions.

| | |
|---|---|
| **Neale Analysis of Reading Ability (NARA)**, second revised British Edition<br>• 6 years–12 years 11 months | Separate norms for accuracy, speed and comprehension yielding standard scores, percentile rank and age equivalents. Two alternate tests enable retesting. |
| **New Reading Analysis**<br>• 7 years 5 months–13 years | Scores for accuracy and comprehension are given in the form of broad range of age equivalents; no standard scores or percentiles. Three sets of passages and record forms for retesting. |

| Diagnostic Reading Analysis (DRA)<br>• 7–16 years | Gives standardised scores for reading accuracy, comprehension, and fluency/reading rate. Parallel forms for retesting. |
| --- | --- |
| Gray Oral Reading Test<br>• 6 years–18 years 11 months | A fluency score is derived from separate rate and accuracy results; all available as standard scores, percentile ranks and age equivalents. Two parallel forms. |

Both the **Revised Neale Analysis** and **New Reading Analysis** are suitable only for the early stages of secondary education, or for readers who are very far behind.

A useful aspect of the **Revised Neale Analysis** is that the results can be compared with those on the **Phonological Ability Battery** (PhAB) and **British Ability Scales** (BAS) for diagnostic purposes (see Chapter 9 of the Neale *Manual for Psychological Services*). Many teachers favour the Neale because it is a less intimidating test than others, since the tester supplies words which are misread or refused by the pupil. Some would also suggest that this makes it a fairer test of text comprehension, whereas others claim the results mislead (Spooner et al 2004).

The **Diagnostic Reading Analysis** is designed for less able readers and incorporates a passage for assessing whether listening comprehension is age-appropriate. The pupil's performance on this part determines the level at which he should start the reading assessment.

The **Gray Oral Reading Test** is American and comprises developmentally sequenced reading passages, each with five comprehension questions in multiple-choice format.

Alternatively, any age-appropriate text can be used to read aloud to the student and probe his comprehension by preparing questions that test both literal and inferential understanding – i.e. not only his ability to recall factual information (*who*, *what*, *where*, *when*, etc), but also his ability to infer from the text.

### ■ Silent reading tests
Silent reading tests, play a useful part in the testing of reading at secondary level. They can be administered as group tests and so they are suitable for screening purposes. Those that are timed are particularly relevant for gauging need for additional time allowances during examinations since they reflect the examination situation quite well.

| Edinburgh Reading Test 4<br>• 11 years 7 months–17 years<br>• timed: 45 minutes | Gives standard score and age equivalent for reading attainment under timed conditions, plus an individual diagnostic profile. |
|---|---|
| Wide Range Achievement Test – Expanded Edition (WRAT-E)<br>Form G; Level 5<br>• 5–18 years<br>• timed: 40 minutes | Results given in standard scores, percentiles and age equivalents. Also includes maths and non-verbal reasoning tests. |
| Vernon-Warden Reading Test<br>• 8 years–adult<br>• timed: 10 minutes | Free to download from the Dyslexia Institute website. Targets comprehension of *sentences* not passages. This is a very old test, so norms may not be accurate. |
| Gray Silent Reading Tests (GSRT)<br>• 7–25 years<br>• untimed | Gives age equivalents, percentiles and a Silent Reading Quotient. Two parallel forms. |

In all these tests, the responses to comprehension questions are by multiple choice and so no writing is involved.

The **Edinburgh Reading Test 4** provides a scoring mechanism for assessing different aspects of reading: skimming, understanding vocabulary, reading for facts and opinions, and inferential comprehension. It therefore provides a comprehensive survey of many of the reading skills needed at Key Stages 3 and 4.

The **Vernon-Warden Reading Test (Revised)** has not been nationally standardised and the content of this test is sometimes old-fashioned. Other tests are preferable.

If administering any of these tests individually, bear in mind the following advice:

> *One aspect to look out for if conducting a comprehension involving silent reading. . . . is to watch the lips of the [learner] while reading to see if they are moving [suggesting] that fast automatised access to the meaning of the passage is still some way off.*

(Beech and Singleton 1997)

### ■ Analysis of reading strategies

A comprehensive profile of a student's individual strategies in a variety of contexts – both single words and continuous text, timed and untimed – should be built up. The fuller the profile, the more easily targets for remediation can be set. Fluency becomes a significant issue in Key Stage 4 as the amount of reading during examination courses increases.

However, it is wise to treat scores with caution. Results of reading tests in particular can be misleading, as different tests do not always compare well with each other. Furthermore, readers may have identical scores but very different strategies and skills. Accuracy scores are based on the number of words read correctly; but the pupil who misreads small words such as *to, of, for* may derive more meaning from the text than the pupil who lacks the word-attack skills to cope with polysyllabic words containing more of the content. Miscue analysis (see page 173) is a useful technique for analysing the reading strategies which lead to errors.

## Writing

While dyslexic pupils may overcome many of their obvious reading difficulties, problems will persist with both quality and quantity of written output. Replicating the writing demands of the classroom in an assessment situation is challenging, and so you should seek out supplementary evidence of the pupil's written work in different subjects, completed independently and preferably under timed conditions.

Assessment should consider writing at word, sentence and text level, in terms of spelling accuracy, legibility and speed of handwriting, as well as overall quality of written output.

The following spelling tests are available for use at secondary level. All can be administered individually or to a group.

| | |
|---|---|
| **Helen Arkell Spelling Test (HAST)**<br>• 5–17 years | Gives percentiles, age-equivalents and standard scores. Designed to be diagnostic. |
| **Wide Range Achievement Test 3 (WRAT–3)** *Spelling*<br>• 5–75 years | Gives standard scores, percentiles and age equivalents: 2 parallel forms (Blue and Tan). Also contains reading and arithmetic tests. |
| **Graded Word Spelling Test**<br>• 6 years–15 years 6 months | Gives standardised scores and age-equivalents. |

In the **HAST** the words represent the normal development of spelling and range from high to low frequency. The test enables the assessor to describe the individual spelling profile and pinpoint a starting point for remediation.

The American **WRAT–3 Spelling Test** is widely used in assessments for access arrangements in public examinations since its norms cover all age groups including 16+. To a certain extent it measures spelling fluency since the instructions are to allow 15 seconds to write each word.

The **Graded Word Spelling Test** is considered by some to be too hard for today's students (Turner 1997).

Single-word spelling can also be checked using lists from the National Literacy Strategy and subject-specific vocabulary lists.

### ■ Analysis of spelling and writing

When analysing spelling, caution should be exercised. Pupils with identical spelling ages may be at different stages of development (see Frith model – page 14). Spelling errors can be 'good' errors (i.e. phonetically acceptable, thus readable) or completely bizarre, with little mapping of letter-sound correspondences. In each case the marks are the same, although remediation and implications for course and exam work would be very different. The timed test from the **Dyslexia Screening Test** can provide a useful measure of spelling ability under timed conditions. As emphasised in previous chapters, it is important to look at the pupil's spelling in free writing.

Free writing is always difficult to assess because its quality depends on many factors, such as the subject matter, about which the student may or may not have much to say! Writing samples should be evaluated qualitatively, in terms of legibility, proportion of words misspelled, proportion of words unreadable and level of vocabulary used. Style, variety and sophistication of sentence structure as well as paragraphing skills should be considered. Dyslexics often have difficulties with organising and sequencing their thoughts and so analysis of the content and structuring of ideas can be at least as, if not more, important to comment on than punctuation and spelling.

However, one issue is of prime importance, given how much writing is expected during this phase of education, and that is speed of writing. This is a crucial issue at Key Stage 4 since the most commonly allowed 'access' arrangement in GCSE exams is extra time to allow for slow writing.

| **Assessment of Handwriting Speed**<br>• 11–16 years<br>• timed: 20 minutes | Timed free-writing task. Continuous prose as in examination conditions. Free from Patoss website. |
|---|---|
| **Sentence Completion Test**<br>• 9–18 years<br>• timed: 10 minutes | Measures writing speed. Less demanding than continuous prose. Free from Dyslexia Institute website. |

At present there are two accepted methods of gauging writing speed:

1   Allcock's **Assessment of Handwriting Speed** is based on research which has been ongoing since 2001. The test uses a 20-minute free-writing task.

This method is described on the Patoss website, where research results are also given.

2 The **Sentence Completion Test** by Hedderly offers a different approach. It can be group administered and has 40 sentences to complete in about 10 minutes. Writing speed can be calculated. An average of 17 words per minute (wpm) at age 15 has been reported. Results may not show difficulty with more able students, as completing a sentence is less demanding than writing continuous prose.

Of interest is the current development of a standardised test by Anna Barnett and Sheila Henderson. It aims to separate out the mechanical aspects of handwriting from other components of expressive writing. Normative data on pupils between the ages of 10 and 16 will be collected in tandem with the re-standardisation of the **Movement Assessment Battery for Children** (M-ABC II). This resource will be published by Harcourt-UK in 2005–6 and should provide a reliable measure of speed of handwriting under different writing conditions.

## Mathematics

| Mathematics Competency Test<br>• 11 years 6 months–18 years | Utilises open-ended questions. Can provide useful information about how an individual's literacy and language skills affect his/her maths learning. |
| --- | --- |

The **Mathematics Competency Test** is suitable for groups or individuals. The instructions can be read to the candidate, but in these circumstances the norms are not then valid, although the test can be used diagnostically. When the learner reads the questions, this test can provide the assessor with useful information about how an individual's literacy and language skills affect his/her maths learning at Key Stages 3 and 4. Learners with weak literacy and/or language skills are likely to have difficulty with:

■ understanding and interpreting questions;

■ matching vocabulary to concepts, formulae and operations;

■ documenting their thinking when writing up investigations.

The questions are similar to those encountered in textbooks, exams and tests. Therefore, as well as identifying specific areas of strength and weakness, the assessor can identify how individuals would cope with the demands they would expect to meet in the maths classroom.

# Cognitive skills

| Phonological Assessment Battery (PhAB)<br>• 6 years–14 years 11 months | The timing component in some subtests means that it can differentiate those pupils for whom automaticity and speed of processing are a problem. |
|---|---|
| Perin Spoonerism Task<br>• Year 10 | Free to download from the Dyslexia Institute website. |
| Comprehensive Test of Phonological Processing (CTOPP)<br>• 5 years–24 years 11 months | A standardised American test which contains many subtests to cover development across this wide age range. |

## Phonological processing

At this stage, assessment of phonological skills tends to be more for diagnosing dyslexia than planning teaching. However, although students may be able to clap or count the largest segments in words – syllables – it is very often the case that they do not know how to apply this skill when spelling longer words. In most cases, they will have developed basic segmentation and blending skills, albeit without ease or fluency. It is the lack of automaticity which holds the key to understanding why literacy skills have not developed as expected and so timed tests are now the most useful.

The **Phonological Assessment Battery (PhAB)** is a standardised test with a ceiling of 14 years and 11 months. It comprises tests of phonological awareness (alliteration and rhyme), fluency (alliteration, rhyme and semantic), semi- and full spoonerisms, and rapid naming (pictures and digits). Spoonerisms and Naming Speed are particularly appropriate for secondary pupils.

The **Comprehensive Test of Phonological Processing (CTOPP)** covers a wide age range and only those most appropriate for an individual student would be used. Composite scores are generated for phonological awareness, phonological memory and rapid naming. Performance in the elision subtest (phoneme deletion) as well as in rapid naming and verbal memory is often revealing in older students.

## Memory

| Working Memory Test Battery for Children (WMTB-C)<br>• 5–15 years | Designed to reflect the Baddley and Hitch 'Working Memory Model' (see page 21). Three measures of central executive, phonological loop and visuo-spatial sketchpad function take about an hour. |
| --- | --- |
| Digit Memory Test<br>• 6 years to adult<br>• timed: 10 minutes | Most widely used method. Free to download from the Dyslexia Institute website. |

Memory is a highly complex skill to assess. It cannot be evaluated in isolation, as it is so affected by other factors such as attention, concentration and levels of anxiety. While a test may claim that it is assessing visual, auditory or motor skills, many pupils will draw on memorising strategies other than those being tested, such as **visualising** letters or numbers in a test of **auditory** recall. It is therefore important to ascertain, by questioning the pupil, what strategies were used. Particularly relevant for dyslexic teenagers are tests which assess working memory and speed of processing.

## Visual/motor skills

| Manual Dexterity Test<br>• 15 years+<br>• timed: 10 minutes | Quick to administer and inexpensive. |
| --- | --- |
| Symbol Digit Modalities Test (SDMT)<br>• 8–17 years | Measures facility with printed symbols and visual-motor speed; takes under 5 minutes. |

The impetus to assess visual/motor skills may well come from concerns about handwriting legibility and speed at this stage.

The Morrisby **Manual Dexterity Test** is useful for demonstrating significant problems with fine motor skills. Norms are available from age 15-plus.

The **Symbol Digit Modalities Test (SDMT)** is similar to the digit symbol coding subtest of the WISC III. It should be used only in conjunction with other tests.

# Feedback and discussion

**Demystification** is an essential part of the assessment procedure at this stage.

Assessment can determine the nature of the learner's problems and often offers labels that are useful for educators. Nevertheless, experience tells us that this on its own may not enable the learner to move forward. He may continue to be confused and disappointed by his own performance, have low self-esteem and believe that poor achievement is his fault.

It is important to explain to each pupil the nature of his learning abilities, his strengths and weaknesses. This can, in turn, empower him to be his own advocate, to devise ways to compensate for or bypass weaknesses, to utilise strengths and value his own individuality. This is the first step to enabling him to work on difficulties with a realistic and positive self-image.

Returning now to Abdul and Susie, the two students described earlier in this chapter: Figures 6.1 and 6.2 show what their assessments indicated and how they will be used to enlighten and help these two young people.

# Modes of intervention

6 *Assessments are only as useful as the interventions that result from them. . . . it is the "so what?" questions that matter. . . . What instructional plans result from the assessment?* 9
(Reid and Wearmouth 2002)

Whilst one might expect the main focus of remediation to be in the realms of study skills, firmly tied into curriculum work, it should be borne in mind that some pupils will still need help at a much more basic level. Poor readers will continue to have difficulty accessing the curriculum, no matter how highly organised they are. Thus specialist teaching may need to prioritise underpinning literacy skills. However, this should, as far as possible, be relevant to the subjects the learner is studying. Revisiting phonics programmes that have been worked on before is likely to alienate an adolescent.

The theme of demystification – fostering the student's clear understanding of his own strengths and difficulties and helping him engage in his own target-setting – was referred to earlier. This is the essence of nurturing metacognitive awareness and is particularly relevant when you are planning an intervention programme.

**Abdul** (age 12 years 6 months)

| Standard Deviation | −3 | −2 | −1  0  +1 | | +2 | +3 |
|---|---|---|---|---|---|---|
| Test | *Well Below* | *Below average* | ← *Average* → *range* | | *Above average* | *Well Above* |
| BPVS | | | X | | | |
| Raven's SPM | | | | X | | |
| Reading – WRAT | | | X | | | |
| NARA – Accuracy | | | X | | | |
| Comprehension | | X | | | | |
| Maths Competency Test | | X | | | | |
| Spelling – WRAT | | | X | | | |
| Rapid naming – pictures – PhAB | | | X | | | |
| Spoonerisms – PhAB | | | X | | | |
| Verbal memory – Digit Span | | X | | | | |

Abdul learns from his assessment that his particular difficulties with mathematics are linked to specific problems with vocabulary, memory and comprehension, although he is quite good at calculation. This means that in class he finds reading and interpreting maths questions difficult. This explanation was meaningful to him as he finds questions involving fractions difficult to understand. Informal probing revealed that he did not know the meaning of *sixth*, *third*, etc. He could demonstrate the correct procedure for working out LCM (lowest common multiple) but didn't know what it all meant. He also said he was not too good at shapes because he could not remember their names.

Multisensory teaching methods will show him how to use all his senses and work more effectively. In particular, his teacher is going to explain maths words and concepts by linking real-life examples to visual (diagrams), verbal and symbolic representations, making sure that Abdul himself does the drawing and writing.

He is reassured that his difficulty is a specific one and that his practical abilities fall within the upper average range. Understanding his own strengths will allow him to utilise his good visuo-spatial ability and enable him to develop his skills in areas of the maths curriculum such as shape and space and graph work which will be important for his career.

His reluctance to read and his dislike of English was unsurprising given his weak comprehension of text. Miscue analysis showed he did not make good use of context cues when reading, so promoting use of 'top down' strategies was recommended in the report.

Figure 6.1

**Susie** (age 16 years)

| Standard Deviation | −3 | −2 | −1   0   +1 | +2 | +3 |
|---|---|---|---|---|---|
| Test | *Well Below* | *Below average* | *← Average → range* | *Above average* | *Well Above* |
| BPVS | | X | | | |
| Raven's SPM | | | X | | |
| Reading – WRAT | | | X | | |
| Sight word efficiency – TOWRE | | X | | | |
| Decoding efficiency – TOWRE | X | | | | |
| Speed/Comprehension (Kirklees) | | X | | | |
| Spelling – HAST | | X | | | |
| Writing speed (Allcock) | | | X | | |
| Rapid naming – pictures – PhAB | X | | | | |
| Spoonerisms – PhAB | X | | | | |
| Verbal memory – Digit Span | | X | | | |

Susie learns from her assessment that she has a sound level of reasoning ability, although her vocabulary is a little weak. Her spelling is generally quite logical. Her handwriting is excellent and so her written work is legible and well presented. Her reading accuracy at word level is sound for her age, but she has difficulty processing verbal information at speed, so her rate of reading is slow. Her difficulties are typical of dyslexia, since the primary problem is with the application of her phonic knowledge. Being taught about syllable division will make a big difference and enable her to tackle longer words when writing. Linked to this will be the development of skills in using an electronic spellchecker effectively.

She will be allowed extra time in her GCSE examinations to compensate for her below-average reading and processing speeds. Her self-esteem and confidence are boosted by her difficulties and worries being acknowledged and understood and by the practical plans for addressing them.

Figure 6.2

❛ *The most valuable and sophisticated ordering of experiences is metacognition – the awareness of your intellectual activities, such as thought processes, concentration and memory, so that they can be used most effectively. Individuals who make use of effective planning and self-monitoring perform better . . . . They can become self-organised and are free to learn from experience.* ❜                (Freeman 2000)

At secondary school students are notoriously disaffected as well as being hypersensitive. Working towards goals imposed by teachers is definitely not 'cool'. Working towards your *own* goals might be just about acceptable, especially when you can see that they relate to your own interests and have an adult slant.

■ **Recommendations** could include targets for:

## Reading fluency and confidence

Paired reading schemes through which older students support Year 7 and 8 children operate successfully in many secondary schools. To access the texts needed for GCSE literature (e.g. novels, plays) get simplified versions; read these first; watch the film/video/play; get the audio version and 'pair read' with the book. Recommend teaching time-effective reference skills for both books and the Internet (e.g. using the index; chapter summaries and so on in books; skimming and scanning techniques in order to get the gist of a text and pick out the salient facts).

## Study skills

Work on note-taking and memory skills; organisation of time, belongings and homework.

## Exam techniques

How to revise – when and where; using notes, card systems and mnemonics; practice with old exam papers; timed questions. Question analysis. Coping with stress.

## Writing

The use of mind maps, time-lines, *Inspiration* writing frames for planning. Focus on multisyllable words in spelling: morphemes; subject-specific vocabulary; use of *spelling* dictionaries; personal spelling memo books or cards; electronic dictionaries and spell-checkers. Encourage word processing for redrafting/editing. Focus on a few useful spelling rules – for suffixing, plurals, etc.

Look at different types of essays; how to build sentences and paragraphs and plan projects. Concentrate on handwriting being legible where possible – if not, go for word processing wherever permissible.

## Memory

Find out how memory works; use different personal strategies for rote learning and revision – visualisation, posters, mind maps, auditory input and multisensory techniques.

## Numeracy

Focus on personal learning style; consolidate knowledge of maths language and number facts and go for bypass strategies like number squares and calculators. Think about how to remember formulae (using memory techniques). Look at ways of improving recording – particularly in longer investigations. Explore and visualise the language of maths. Look for examples from a real context. Draw or sketch maths problems.

## Summary

- Particular difficulties arise at the secondary stage because of the more fragmented nature of the curriculum and its increasing demands on higher-level literacy skills.
- Some students continue to experience difficulties at a basic level which subject teachers are not really trained to deal with.
- Others find that the increasing demands of the curriculum present challenges to their study and organisation skills, as well as their ability to read and write fluently.
- Examinations become a major concern.
- Self-esteem is often fragile.
- Appropriate assessment resources cover many of the same areas as at the primary stage – but they must be age-appropriate and relate to the skills needed at this stage.
- The student himself is a primary source of information at this stage. He must be an active partner in both the assessment and in setting targets.
- The aim is for him, as well as his teachers and parents, to have a clearer picture of his strengths, difficulties and best ways of working.

# 7 Further and Higher Education

## Further Education

Kath Morris and Annie White

This section looks at:

- the varied needs and expectations of students in further education;

- how students with needs for additional learning support can be identified through initial screening and (where necessary) full diagnostic assessment;

- planning for appropriate teaching programmes.

People-watching in a crowded college refectory during a typical lunchtime is a fascinating experience. The queue for the salads and sandwiches bar usually includes a small group of girls from the Health and Beauty or Hairdressing courses, easily identified by their tight-fitting white uniform and elaborate make-up. Most of them are fresh out of school, but there will also be one or two who are fresh out of domesticity and child-rearing. Further down the queue is a small group of much older people who have paid their dues in respect of raising children and undertaking gainful employment and are now enjoying their leisure time by learning how to paint. Finally, there is a member of the administrative staff who spends the larger part of her college life creating order out of chaos for a Senior Manager and a smaller (but significant) part as a student on a FENTO[7] Train to Teach course based at the college. She has decided she would like to try her hand at passing on some of the valuable knowledge she has acquired in her own specialist field.

On the other side of the cash tills, queuing for hot meals, is an equally varied cross-section of the population. First in the queue are the gas engineers who are well established in their chosen careers and have come on a short course to update their CORGI registrations. Many of these students left school with no academic qualifications at all and learned their trade as apprentices. Jostling for position, just behind them, are the Travel and Tourism students. This is a mixed group. Some of these students performed well at GCSE level; some fared slightly worse but are hoping for a new start because they are finally motivated to learn; and some are definitely 'only here for the beer'.

---

[7] FENTO: Further Education National Training Organisation.

Tucked into a corner with their home-packed lunches is a group of students on the Access to Higher Education course who are engaged in an animated discussion relating to that morning's lecture. Some of these students will have gained reasonable grades at A-level in the recent past and some (like the gas engineers) will have no formal qualifications at all. Many of them will have dropped out of formal education at the first opportunity, having been totally demoralised by critical teachers. They are now returning to fulfil a dream of receiving a 'decent' education, often having gained confidence in their own abilities either by successfully rearing children or by successfully starting up a business.

This is a diverse group of diners with diverse educational needs. The only common ground is that they are all enrolled as students in the same College of Further Education.

## *The FE environment*

Those working in this wonderfully diverse world will need to know the territory. Many features of the terrain will seem unfamiliar to those more used to other sectors of education. This applies particularly to provision for special educational needs (including dyslexia).

To begin with, the terminology is different. In FE, 'Students with Learning Difficulties and Disabilities' (SLDD) has been the term used to replace 'Students with SEN' since 1992, when the FE/HE Act ended the role of the Local Education Authorities in further education. SLDD is an umbrella term that includes specific learning difficulties such as dyslexia.

Funding arrangements are also different from those in both schools and higher education. The Further Education Funding Council (FEFC) was established under the terms of the 1992 Act and has subsequently been replaced by the Learning and Skills Council (LSC). This huge funding body has, as part of its remit, the funding of provision for SLDD. Currently, Additional Learning Support (ALS) in FE is funded by the LSC via the Additional Learning Funding Mechanism. Provision of funding is based on evidence of need which individual colleges must document meticulously in their claims. This requirement for hard evidence, along with the underlying responsibilities placed on all educational bodies – following the Disability Discrimination Act (DDA) in 1995 and the Special Educational Needs and Disability Act (SENDA) in 2001 – obviously drives the need for careful initial screening and assessment.

It is important to note that LSC funding comes to colleges, not individuals. There are no individual grants to students to provide them with support or ICT equipment or software, as there are through the DSA grants awarded by the DfES in higher education. (The exception would be those students on the Access to Higher Education courses.)

The other side of the coin is that the *need* referred to above does not necessarily have to have a label. Students in FE do not have to be proved 'dyslexic' to qualify for support, although dyslexia will clearly be a major underlying factor. For example, the need may be for the services of an amanuensis. The student involved may have a severe physical disability, may be highly intelligent but have totally illegible handwriting, or may sit at the other end of the ability scale and produce such bizarre spellings that no one can decipher them. Each of them will be better able to achieve his individual potential with this form of support.

The strict Code of Practice that applies in schools and sets a staged route – from identification, through school action to statutory assessment – does not apply. Students in FE colleges are more likely to be adults and less likely to have a documented history of need. Many received their schooling long before dyslexia was recognised. Furthermore, many of them will be participating in very part-time courses. Consequently, there will be less time to observe and investigate their needs. For all these reasons, the sooner the identification of need takes place, the better. The ideal would be for all students to be screened for potential need in the first week of their college courses.

# Initial screening

Historically, the screening process in FE colleges involved a paper-based assessment of literacy and numeracy skills. In many colleges, such tests have now been replaced with computerised packages that offer a baseline assessment of these skills. There are also computerised screening programmes that purport to identify those students who are likely to be dyslexic. The advantage of such tests is that they are relatively quick to administer, the analysis is done for you and the findings often come in a printout form. However, we have already discussed the fact that we are not necessarily looking for a *label* of dyslexia in the FE setting: we are seeking to identify individual needs. In this respect, these computerised packages may not give us the detailed information that we need.

Many students are attracted to FE colleges because they have not fared too well in academic subjects at school. Spelling and grammar may not be their strong points. Their talents are more likely to include an ability to detect a badly tuned engine from the other side of the car park or an ability to spot an ideal composition for a photograph. Students such as these will be hoping to start the next phase of their education with a clean slate, often claiming to have 'forgotten' how many passes (or what grades) they achieved at GCSE level. Their hopes will quickly be dashed if they are subjected to an insensitive assessment of their literacy and numeracy skills within the first few days of college.

What follows is a suggested format for screening these vulnerable students in a way that will not patronise their more academic peers (an equally valid consideration). This assessment will yield valuable data as to the students' individual strengths and difficulties, learning styles and any coping strategies that are already in place. Students are screened in their subject groups as part of the induction process. Where groups are over fifteen in number, it may be better to split them into two smaller groups. The complete assessment takes approximately two hours.

## Note-taking skills

This is a good place to start, as everyone accepts that taking good notes is a required study skill. The assessor introduces herself to the group. Ideally, she will be a member of the college support team and will include an overview of the service as part of this. The students are asked to take notes during this introductory speech. No overheads or handouts are provided and the assessor delivers at a normal talking speed. There is an added advantage to this exercise, in so far as the students are forced to focus upon what is being said. Otherwise, they are likely to stare out of the window in the hope of catching a glimpse of whichever member of the opposite sex has taken their fancy in the last twenty-four hours.

Five minutes on this exercise is quite sufficient. At the end of this time, ask the students to look back over their notes and assess whether or not they would be able to make sense of them in six months' time. Stress that it is only important that *they* can make sense of them; no one else is going to judge them. Take this self-evaluation exercise a little further by encouraging the students to either record the fact that taking notes is something they find relatively easy, or that this is something that they have always found difficult. Ask them to detail any strategies they have developed to help them cope. For example, a student may have a close friend on the same course who has agreed to take notes that can be photocopied.

## Reading

Standardised reading tests often focus on the assessment of reading accuracy. However, there are two further elements to this skill that are often overlooked in the screening process: reading speed and reading comprehension. All elements can be assessed quite neatly using a specially prepared cloze exercise.

Select a short, straightforward passage from one of the course texts (about 200 words should suffice). Copy out the first sentence in its entirety then, in the following sentences, delete approximately every sixth word. Try to ensure that the deleted words include nouns, verbs and adjectives as well as the occasional *and*, *the* or *it*. This will be time-consuming to begin with, but the same passage can then be used over and over again in the future. Ask a colleague or a second-year student to complete the exercise (to fill in the gaps) and record the time taken. Completing comfortably in 10 minutes is a good target. Allow this amount of time for the screening task.

At the end of the set time, ask the students to evaluate their performances. There will be those who found the whole thing very straightforward and completed well within the time limit. These students should record that their reading skills are within the range expected for their level of study. Many find this knowledge very reassuring.

Then there will be a group who managed to think of an appropriate word for each gap but who ran out of time. These students should record the fact that they need to allow extra time for reading tasks. This group may require further (standardised) assessment of their reading speeds with a view to requesting extra time in examinations.

Finally, there will be a group who finished well within the time but who left lots of gaps unfilled. This will be the group with the greatest need, as they will undoubtedly find course texts beyond their comprehension. This group should record that they *'don't always understand text on the first reading.'* Note that no one is asked to record that they have *'a reading difficulty'* as students rarely perceive themselves as being in this category, even when they clearly are. As long as they can decode most of the words on the page, they consider themselves able to read. Unfortunately, none of that is of any use without the attendant comprehension skills.

Once again, students should be encouraged to detail any coping strategies that they have. For example, some students ask a girlfriend to read the text to them so that they can focus on the meaning. If they have already devised strategies that work for them, then they should be given credit for this.

If the problem is really serious, this student may require further, standardised assessment with a view to providing a reader in examinations.

## Spelling and punctuation

Standardised spelling tests assess whether the level of spelling is age-appropriate, but the listed spellings are not necessarily those that the students will require for their course. They may get by in life without ever knowing how many *c*'s and *s*'s there are in *necessary* or when to use the correct form of *practice/practise*. However, it *is* important for a student of Travel and Tourism to be able to spell *tourism*. This should never be taken for granted.

One way to assess relevant spelling skills is to select a short passage from one of the course texts that incorporates some subject-specific vocabulary. Those who are familiar with the subject area will be able to create their own passages to ensure maximum coverage. Fifty words should suffice. The important thing is that the students will accept that these are words they will be expected to spell correctly on a regular basis.

Read the passage through once at normal speed then dictate in small chunks (three to four words at a time) at a pace to accommodate the slowest writer. Read through at normal speed again. On the first and third readings, make it quite clear where one sentence ends and another begins so that very basic punctuation can be checked at the same time. Lists can be included to check knowledge of the use of commas.

As before, ask the students to reflect on their own performances. If they feel they have done reasonably well, then this is what they record. If they know that spelling is a problem, then this is recorded. In the latter case, ask for details of what strategies the students use to tackle unknown words. These may include writing the word as it sounds, getting a girlfriend to proofread coursework before final drafting or always using a word processor with a spell-check function. A student who has such strategies in place may not require any further support. On the other hand, anyone who feels that they would like help in this area can make a note of that fact.

The beauty of this method of assessment is that everything is dealt with in the strictest confidence. At the end of each exercise, *everyone* writes something, not just the ones who found it difficult.

## Summarising

This is the area where most students experience difficulty. Many of those who gained relatively good grades at GCSE will have largely done so without ever mastering this skill.

The best resource for this exercise will be an article from a recent newspaper or magazine on a subject-related topic. For example, students on a Health and Social Care course could be presented with an article on obesity. The article should not be too lengthy and the underlying message should be clear. Before presenting the article to the students, the assessor should check that *she* is able to summarise it in three short sentences within ten to fifteen minutes, using her own words. This is the task that is then set for the students.

Once again, the task is followed by a few minutes of self-evaluation. The students tend to fall into one of three categories. The first will be made up of those who went through the passage with a highlighter and then copied three of these sentences verbatim for their summary. These students should record that they find it difficult to translate texts into their own words.

The second group will have used their own words but will have written a summary that is only marginally shorter than the original article. This group should record that they do not fully understand the concept of summarising and would appreciate some guidance. Note the careful phrasing. It is much easier to admit that something isn't *fully understood* than it is to admit that something is *not known*.

Finally, there will be a group of students who knew exactly what they had to do but who ran out of time. There may even be the odd one or two who achieved the desired outcome within the time frame – these are rare birds and should be cherished as such. Those who ran out of time need to make a note to allow lots of time for such activities when planning their assignment timetables.

## Brainstorming/mind-mapping

Many of the students will have found the assessment to date quite taxing; the following exercise should help to release some of the tension.

The assessor needs to decide on a topic in advance and write this in the centre of the board. The topic does not need to be course-related. 'Parents Know Best!' is usually guaranteed to provoke a response from even the most reticent student. The concept of mind-mapping should then be explained. Most students are familiar with it but may know it by another name. The assessor then offers to act as scribe and tries to create order out of the mayhem that ensues. There will be dominant members of the group; others will say nothing. This is their choice.

Fifteen minutes should be allowed for this exercise before the usual self-evaluation is requested.

On this occasion, the students should reflect upon whether they preferred this group activity to the individual tasks. Those who feel this way should identify other members in the group who feel the same way and set up their own study group to discuss issues before attempting assignments. Those who do not feel this way should be encouraged to reflect upon how they might develop their confidence in public speaking as it will, almost certainly, form part of the assessment process.

## And finally . . .

The assessor asks the students to look back on their school careers and focus on one subject that they enjoyed. Mature students can do this just as easily as recent school-leavers. They are asked to reflect upon what it was that made the learning so easy and the teaching so memorable.

Everything that has been produced in the assessment session is then handed in. It is important that everything is named, as all this information will then be summarised for the course tutors. These summaries will then be discussed in confidence at the first one-to-one tutorials where individual learning plans are drawn up. Students who have identified existing coping strategies should be praised and those who have identified areas where they would like support should have these needs addressed.

# Detailed assessment

Those students who have highlighted concerns in several areas may choose the option of a further, in-depth diagnostic assessment, particularly if the provision of readers, scribes and extra time comes into the equation. The later section on assessment in HE contains helpful guidelines relating to the structure of this more detailed assessment. The following is additional information relating specifically to the world of FE.

Remember the spread of ability and attainment in FE is even wider than it is within HE. Whilst your assessments might cover students at graduate level and above (see Figure 7.1), at the other extreme you might also be asked to assess someone who is working at Entry Level 1 in the Adult Literacy Core Curriculum (Basic Skills Agency 2001). It is not unusual to meet students who, for one reason or another, have extremely limited literacy skills. Be prepared for this and spare them the humiliation of being asked to do something beyond their capabilities. For instance, to ask them to produce timed writing on a given topic will be a complete non-starter – a far better approach would be to ask what things they *can* write. Maybe this will be a job-related task or a greeting on a Christmas card. In order to plan steps forward, the comfortable follow-up from this is to ask what they would like to *be able to* write.

In the case of most FE students, background information should be gathered by discussion. Many of them do not have the confidence to complete a questionnaire independently. Questions along the lines of '*Many people find it difficult to organise their thoughts on paper – would you say that applied to you?*' are more conducive to an honest discussion than '*Do you have a problem organising your ideas?*' It is such a subtle distinction, but it can make all the difference in the world to a nervous student who may be grateful to know that he is not on his own.

Of particular importance is the need to allow time at the end of the assessment for a discussion of all that has taken place. Ideally, the student should also be invited to a follow-up session, once the report has been prepared, so that they have a chance to read through before it is passed to other interested parties. This is not always possible in the real world, so a compromise might be to send out the report with a covering letter to the student. This letter would contain a succinct summary of the findings in very clear language.

# Teaching programmes

The guidelines relating to writing teaching programmes that are set out in Chapter 8 can also be applied at FE level, but with one or two caveats. The following are issues to be considered. First and foremost there is the issue of whether a teaching programme is required at all. The screening process will galvanise some students into requesting an in-depth assessment to provide the

**Chloe** (aged 24)

Chloe referred herself for assessment. She is a graduate now studying for an NVQ in Advice and Guidance, with a view to working in careers guidance. Whilst feeling confident in her ability to express her opinions articulately, she doesn't feel that she is doing herself justice on paper in her studies. She suspects that she might be dyslexic and there is a family history of such difficulties, but she has never been formally assessed or had any previous learning support.

Assessment showed that Chloe has an excellent vocabulary and an average level of non-verbal skills. Whereas her reading at single-word level was in the average range, both comprehension skills and speed of reading were below average. In addition the reading process was very tiring for her – she described reading as being like *'looking through dirty glass'*. A rather similar mismatch showed in assessment of her writing skills: whilst the content was appropriate to her level of study, Chloe's writing speed was below average. Her spelling was in the average range, but she confided that when writing by hand she would always play safe and use only those words that she knew how to spell correctly. When word-processing she would rely on the spell-check to pick up errors and be more adventurous. Embarrassment about spelling worried Chloe – she felt frightened of making mistakes in a 'public' situation and her lecture notes were sparse as she spent a great deal of time thinking how to rephrase what was being said. A Digit Span memory test suggested that Chloe's memory skills were well below average.

Chloe is an intelligent, articulate young woman who achieved good results both at school and at university: one would expect test results to reflect that. Her single-word reading and spelling test results put her in the 'average' band of the population. However, Chloe is not average.

Did the assessment help her? Chloe now has a better understanding of her difficulties. She can feel a little more confident about her spelling, knowing that it is at least at the same level as the majority of the population of her age. She has been encouraged to take risks in her spelling – particularly in examinations – and is now aware that the few marks she will sacrifice because of any misspelled words will easily be made up if she completes more questions and writes in a more sophisticated style.

Her assessor was able to discuss strategies with Chloe for helping with other difficulties such as the development of her own 'shorthand' for taking notes, both in lectures and from course textbooks. She is interested in adopting memory strategies – such as visualising a very large nail or hook on the far side of the room on which to 'hang' a conversation until it becomes necessary to retrieve it: she thought this would help her focus on the main threads in an interview or discussion. She is prepared to discuss her difficulties with her tutors and will seek help from a Behavioural Optometrist specialising in visual difficulties and dyslexia.

**Figure 7.1**

necessary evidence for Additional Learning Support. They will accept that the time has finally come to address the issues of spelling or time-management. These students will require teaching programmes.

There will be other students who request an in-depth assessment more to satisfy an inner curiosity as to why it was that they fared so badly at school, despite a sneaking suspicion that they were at least as bright as their higher achieving peers. The members of this group are just seeking an explanation and an opportunity to discuss all that has been suppressed over the years. They will not necessarily need teaching recommendations as well. The example of Chloe (Figure 7.1) fits into this category. The recommendations made are for Chloe – to help her manage her learning better and help her to become more independent.

For those who do need individual teaching programmes, the emphasis may well be on work at the sentence and text level rather than word level. The content of the programme is more likely to be weighted towards study skills, reading comprehension, assignment planning and exam preparation. Any word-level work is more likely to be based on mastering subject vocabulary rather than a structured phonics programme.

There are national standards for adult literacy[8] but the targets for writing, even at the basic level, focus on the ability to communicate information *'with some awareness of the intended audience'*. There is no target for being able to spell a given list of words, as there is in the primary school classroom. The learning support tutor in FE will often find herself in a situation where she is supporting at two levels. The student may well be on an A-level Sociology course with literacy skills more akin to those of a nine-year-old. The tutor must put aside the fact that he cannot always spell *said* correctly and focus on keeping him up to date with his coursework.

Targets can (and should) still be **SMART** but with a slightly different emphasis – as follows:

**S**pecific: what will the student be able to do by the end of the teaching programme? For example: Jess will learn how to use the program *Inspiration* to produce mind maps for planning her Health and Social Care assignments.

**M**easurable: how will the student demonstrate he/she can do what is required? Jess will explain the program to another student without any input from the tutor.

---

[8] The National Standards for Adult Literacy and Numeracy, DfES website: http://www.dfes.gov.uk/curriculum_literacy/intro/ns/

**A**chievable: is this a realistic target for six weeks' work? Might it be more realistic to set a target of simply producing one mind map to cover one assignment? Alternatively, might it be possible for Jess to demonstrate to her entire course-group using Powerpoint?

**R**elevant: Jess needs to be able to plan her work. She wants to get good grades in her assignments. The fact that she is using ICT means that she can simultaneously use the spell-check facility to help with the subject vocabulary that she frequently misspells.

**T**ime-related: it is important that Jess gets to grips with this software quickly. She is falling behind. She must have mastered the technique by week 6.

It is of paramount importance that all targets are negotiated with the student. The above illustration involved only one target. Jess may well have others. She may also need to use the technique to produce (with assistance in the early stages) plans for two assignments. She may need to have produced a timetable for revision for her mock examinations; she may need to devise a set of icons to help her take notes more effectively in her lectures; she may even express a wish to be able to spell *psychology* reliably, etc.

It is also important for the student to be involved in the continual process of evaluation as to whether or not the programme is effective and appropriate. Checking for mastery is less likely to be done by tests and dictations and more likely to involve production of coursework.

As regards *methods* and *resources*, it is vital that these are appropriate to both the student's age and his/her preferred learning style. Jess may be perfectly happy to use a salt tray to learn her spelling; another student might not be. The *pace* of teaching is always an important consideration, and with older students there is the added complication of fitting in with ridiculously tight teaching schedules and weeks out of college on work experience.

## Summary

- The population of a typical FE college is one of considerable diversity in terms of the range of age, ability and educational experience.
- Funding for Additional Learning Support goes to the college rather than the student. Funding is available only where there is clear evidence of need. The need does not have to have the label *dyslexia*.
- This need has to be identified at the earliest opportunity. Comprehensive screening of *all* new students is just as important as in-depth diagnostic assessment of a much smaller number.
- Any programmes resulting from these in-depth assessments must be negotiated with the student and delivered in age-appropriate ways.

# Higher Education      Katherine Kindersley

'New opportunities are unfolding that may require special talents and abilities in just those areas where many individuals with learning difficulties often have their greatest strengths. Different kinds of problems and different kinds of tools may require different kinds of talents and favour different kinds of brains.'

(West 1991)

## *Particular considerations for students in Higher Education*

- The Special Educational Needs and Disability Act (SENDA) requires Higher Education institutions to make reasonable adjustments to enable students with dyslexia and other forms of specific learning difficulty (SpLD) to access the curriculum and demonstrate achievement of learning outcomes. Such provision and the availability of support through the Disabled Students' Allowance (DSA) encourages students with difficulties to come forward for assessment.

- Many students are identified with specific learning difficulties for the first time at HE level. The increased level of study demands, including higher-order language use, as well as the need for greater independence in learning and in the organisation of study, can reveal problems which may go unnoticed in the more structured school environment, or may be masked by an enormous amount of effort on the pupil's part.

- Increasingly schools have tried to move away from labelling students, seeking rather to identify their strengths, so that these can be exploited, and their weaknesses, which can be supported. This remains the guiding principle of all those involved in assessment at HE level, but if students are to receive funding under the DSA, a specific diagnostic label is also required. Moreover, without this label, students who have received additional time in GCSE and A-level examinations may not be considered eligible for the same arrangements at university level.

- The world of HE is a varied one, and HE students are a very heterogeneous group, in terms of age, educational background and academic qualifications. A student may arrive with A-levels straight from school or be a pensioner who has decided to embark on a course at the Open University. Many mature students may well have attended Access Courses. Widening participation means that some students are embarking on degree courses having received little in the way of formal training for essay writing, or coping with academic text. Assessment may reveal that dyslexia is not the cause of their problems with academic study, but lack of study skills teaching is a factor. Fortunately, in many universities, there is increasing study support within the institution for those who need it, yet who fall outside the DSA provision.

■ More problematic is where assessment reveals an even, below-average test profile and the presence of general learning difficulties. Sensitive advice needs to be given, if possible in liaison with the institution's support officers and combined with effective careers guidance.

■ For the purposes of applying for DSA funding, a student identified as having dyslexia before the age of 16 years may only require an 'Assessment of Performance Attainment', a 'top-up' diagnosis to establish the likely impact of his specific learning difficulties on the skills needed for higher education. However, some LEAs require a full diagnostic assessment to be completed at the tertiary stage.

■ The written reports for HE students can be expected to have a number of quite different audiences: the student, the Disability Advisor or Dyslexia Coordinator, the student's tutors or supervisors, examination and assessment officers, the specialist support tutor, the LEA officers. The reports therefore have a range of purposes and these must be kept in mind.

■ As far as possible, tests should be standardised on the adult population. It is inappropriate to report test ages.

■ According to proposals under consideration by the DfES, those assessing students for DSA purposes will have to hold a Current Practising Certificate in SpLD Assessment, regularly updated (DfES National SpLD Assessment Framework: see DfES website).

## *Indicators of difficulties*

There can be many reasons for seeking an assessment. Students may be alerted to their difficulties by tutors, by talking to fellow students or by their own struggle to meet course demands. Awareness may also be raised by Disability Officers and through induction talks. Others have been aware for many years of the great effort they must make with aspects of learning, but have not had opportunities for assessment.

It should be recognised that, at HE level, many students have compensated for their literacy difficulties and may perform adequately on tests of single-word reading and spelling accuracy. They do, however, encounter problems with more subtle and complex aspects of written language, and such difficulties are exacerbated when demands are made on their memory and organisational skills, as well as their ability to process information at speed.

Students can study a plethora of subjects at degree level and the nature of the demands on the student will vary according to his course. The specific manifestations of difficulty will therefore be equally varied, but students' concerns are likely to be in the following areas:

- **Reading** speed and comprehension. Despite the fact that many students read for pleasure, having perfected a skim reading and prediction strategy, a recurring theme is the time it takes them to read and comprehend academic text, because they have been unable to develop additional reading strategies for different types of text. There may also be visual disturbance when reading, or concerns about misreading words, particularly under time pressure, as well as a horror of reading aloud in tutorials and seminars.

- **Writing skills:** organising language and structuring ideas in written work. Even if sentence structure and paragraphing skills are sound, students may still be overwhelmed by the sheer volume and complexity of thoughts to be organised. Such students often turn in excellent course work, but this is the product of many drafts and repeated revision, and the individual is therefore at a disadvantage in examinations, where redrafting is not an option.

- **Spelling.** Spelling skills often fragment under pressure. In exams, anxiety about spelling may lead students to restructure their sentences in order to avoid problem words, or to use less appropriate ones, which disrupts writing fluency considerably.

- **Spoken language.** Students having problems with producing written work may also experience difficulty with expressive language, feeling that they cannot express their ideas adequately. As a result, they contribute as little as possible in seminars, and dread verbal presentations.

- **Memory and organisation.** Students may struggle to remember names and numbers, and to master unfamiliar academic/technical terms. Mental calculation is slow and effortful and they have problems dealing with strictly sequenced material, such as an alphabetical index. Such problems frequently compromise the ability to follow lectures and take effective notes. Weaknesses in organisation often show up in difficulties with time management, missing appointments/deadlines, managing and prioritising the very varied and multilayered demands of some courses, as well as balancing study and home life.

- **Other difficulties.** There may be additional difficulties with aspects of visual perception, visuo-motor tasks and coordination.

# Ways of assessing

Adequate time must be allowed for the assessment. All assessments should be conducted in a patient and sensitive manner, but adult students – especially those being assessed for the first time – are likely to have questions which need to be answered and fears which need to be allayed before and during the course of the assessment. A screening assessment may have already probed sensitive areas, highlighting earlier unhappy experiences, contributing to the emotional impact of the assessment. Time should also be allowed for some immediate feedback at the end of the assessment session, and assessors need to communicate this information sensitively in order to help students accept the results. While it can often be a relief for students to know that there is a recognised cause for their difficulties, some will have misgivings about labels. The assessor can help by explaining the outcome in terms of differences in learning style, by highlighting the student's strengths and discussing how these can be exploited in the learning process.

# Collecting background information

It is important to take a proper background history. This may be gathered partly via a questionnaire completed before the assessment, or alternatively through a series of structured questions and discussion during the assessment. Such discussion gives insight into the student's main concerns, the purpose of the assessment and how the student can be helped. It may be that information taken at a screening procedure, can, with the student's permission, be forwarded to the assessor.

Information should be gathered on the following, and the quality of oral explanations should be noted:

## Family history

Are any other family members affected by difficulties with written and/or spoken language?

## General health

Vision and hearing – have these been checked? Eliminate the obvious. Is general health good, or is there anything which might have a bearing on the student's current difficulties?

## Speech and language

Check whether the student received speech therapy, and whether he recalls any problems with spoken language in the early years. Is he prone to word-finding difficulties, mispronunciations or word confusions now?

### Motor development

Was he considered to be a clumsy child? Did handwriting skills develop slowly? How is his fine and gross coordination now? Persistent motor coordination problems can indicate the presence of DCD (dyspraxia).

### Educational history

Were literacy skills slow to develop? Was additional support received at any stage? Check GCSE and A-level results, if appropriate.

### School experience

Were difficulties handled sensitively, or was the student humiliated or ignored? Did he feel able to access all areas of the curriculum? Were there frequent changes of school? Did the student have prolonged periods of absence or truanting?

### Current difficulties

Explore current difficulties fully, including questions about tutor feedback (see indicators of difficulties, above).

## Observation

Since the student may have developed effective compensatory strategies, certain difficulties can be hard to detect. Careful observation during testing is, therefore, crucial, in order to produce an accurate assessment. There is, for example, a world of difference between two students who score 105 on a standardised spelling test, one with apparent ease, the other by thinking long and hard about each word, with multiple attempts. Similarly, circumlocutions and hesitations do not show up in final scores, yet will undoubtedly be related to difficulties with writing. Are there indicators of visual perceptual difficulties when reading, such as omission or repetition of lines, or does the student finger-track? Are working memory measures and/or phonological measures accompanied by a huge amount of effort, and possibly hand movement, which suggests the processing involved is a strain? It may be appropriate to use test behaviour as evidence of a difficulty when standardised scores belie the effort the students put into tasks.

## Formal and informal tests

There is an increasing range of appropriate tests available to the specialist teacher assessor. Updated lists are available in the DfES National Assessment Framework (see DfES website, www.dfes.gov.uk), where a report format is also given.

Assessment should include the following:

- **Measures of literacy attainment:** Single-word reading. Non-word reading. Continuous text reading, oral and silent. Reading speed and reading comprehension. Single-word spelling. Timed free writing. In addition, a copying speed test and a précis writing exercise are useful discriminating measures. (See next section: Interpretation – Measures of Literacy Attainment.)

- **Assessment of general intellectual ability**, with measures of verbal and non-verbal ability.

- **Cognitive processing:** an assessment of adult dyslexia/dyspraxia must include measures of underlying cognitive processes, such as phonological skills, working memory, speed of processing. Difficulties here are common to students with SpLD.

- **Other areas:** it may well be that a student has been referred because of suspected dyslexia, but the assessor should be alert to the possibility of the presence of other SpLDs. For example, perceptual, spatial, motor and coordination difficulties may indicate the presence of DCD/dyspraxia, and sometimes different conditions can co-exist.

If a student reports visual disturbance when reading, it may be appropriate to screen for Meares Irlen Syndrome or to recommend that the student's visual functioning is investigated further, for example by the Institute of Optometry.

Students may initially be apprehensive and the ordering of tests therefore requires careful thought. Vary and pace the type of task to maintain maximum performance.

# Interpretation

## Measures of literacy attainment

Single-word reading can be assessed using the **Wide Range Achievement Test 3** (WRAT–3). Note whether reading rate slows markedly as the student works through the test. How efficiently are letters mapped to sounds, and how easily can the student pronounce polysyllabic words? Note that when students have English as an additional language, it is unwise to record vowel misreadings as errors.

The **Test of Word Reading Efficiency** (TOWRE) assesses word and non-word reading under timed conditions. This is critically important, because it is often only under timed conditions that inefficiencies in the mechanics of reading are revealed. Timed oral reading of continuous text can reveal useful information about the student's reading fluency, and a number of tests such as the **Gray Oral Reading Test** (GORT–4), the **Spadafore Diagnostic Reading Test** (SDRT), or the **Adult Reading Test** (ART), provide appropriate oral reading material. A standardised measure of reading comprehension – using tests such as the **Wide Range Achievement Test–Expanded** (WRAT–E), **Individual Assessment, Form 1, Reading Comprehension Test** or the **Gray Silent Reading Test** (GSRT) – provides necessary information about the student's ability to extract meaning from text. The WRAT–E also provides written language, listening comprehension and oral expression measures.

Single-word spelling accuracy can be assessed using the WRAT–3. Note whether the student relies extensively on sound-letter translation and whether this is reliable; note also whether correctly spelled words are produced instantly, or are the result of several attempts. At HE level, many students will be able to produce reasonable phonetic approximations, but some may rely on a hazy recall of a word's visual appearance and as a result produce rather 'bizarre' spellings.

A copying speed test has been found to be a powerful discriminator in identifying students with dyslexia at this level, and a timed précis writing exercise provides useful information about the student's ability to manage language and organise a written response to text (Hatcher et al 2002). This research has been used to develop a battery of diagnostic tests, with normative data from the University of York, in the **York Adult Assessment Battery** (YAA).

An informal but crucial test is a timed piece of free writing. The student's ability to communicate ideas, and to structure and organise these at sentence level and in the overall piece, should be noted, as well as his ability to spell in context, to use vocabulary effectively, and to retain grammatical and technical accuracy. Handwriting speed and legibility should also be recorded, in order to inform decisions about examination arrangements.

## Intellectual ability

The **Wide Range Intelligence Test** (WRIT) provides a powerful and sensitive measure of intellectual ability. It gives a general IQ from four factors which correlate in a 'nearly indistinguishable way' with the comparable factors in the **Weschler Adult Intelligence Scale**.

The pattern of scores should be noted, particularly any significant difference between verbal and non-verbal ability. If a student's problems with aspects of expressive language appear to compromise their performance on the vocabulary scale, it is worth administering a test of receptive vocabulary such as the **Peabody Picture Vocabulary Test**. The PPVT-III measures vocabulary in the same way as the **British Picture Vocabulary Test** (BPVS-II), but the advantage of the former is that it provides norms up to 90 years, whereas the BPVS has a ceiling of 15 years and relies on a much smaller sample of adults (150) for those over 16 years.

## Cognitive processing

The **Comprehensive Test of Phonological Processing** (CToPP) taps into different aspects of phonological processing, including processing speed, with its tests of phonological awareness, phonological memory and rapid naming. The Nonsense Passage reading and the Spoonerisms tests from the **York Adult Assessment Battery** may also highlight underlying problems, especially in students at HE level who can perform reasonably well on measures of phonological awareness.

The **Symbol Digit Modalities Test** provides a standardised measure of visuo-motor processing speed, and a discrepancy between visuo-motor speed and broader visuo-spatial reasoning (see WRIT, above) is frequently observed in specific learning difficulties.

A Digit Span test, such as that devised by Ridsdale and Turner of the Dyslexia Institute (2002), provides a standardised measure of auditory short-term and working memory, and is a critical element in the assessment battery. A weakness in working memory, particularly a discrepancy between working memory and verbal ability (see WRIT above), is a reliable indicator of specific learning difficulties. There is also an excellent range of memory tests in the **Wide Range Assessment of Memory and Learning** (WRAML–2), with six core tests providing verbal, visual and attention-concentration indexes. Subtests include sentence memory as well as verbal and symbolic working memory tests.

## Further comments on interpretation

It is in the interpretation of the tests that the skill of the assessor becomes apparent. Testing involves scores and norms, but these have to be interwoven with the other strands of evidence in order to present a coherent picture of the whole person, with his complex mix of strengths and weaknesses.

Ideally, all students should be tested in their first language, but when this is not possible, the results of verbal measures must be interpreted with caution. Moreover, if students consistently mispronounce or confuse particular sounds in their speech, then this will affect how they deal with those sounds in reading and spelling; vowel pronunciation can be particularly vulnerable when English is not the student's first language. These factors need to be taken into account, particularly in timed measures, such as the TOWRE.

### Possible involvement of other professionals

The ideal situation is one in which the assessor works closely with the relevant university staff and accepts referrals through them. The assessor will be knowledgeable about the support (academic and counselling) and accommodations available in the institution and can give specific guidance as to how the student can access these. The assessor also needs to be aware of data protection issues, and where he/she works independently it is essential to ensure that the student gives permission for information disclosure.

# Modes of intervention

The gap between what the student is able to do and what is expected of him on his particular course needs to be made clear, and any recommendations have to take into account the demands being made upon the student if the assessment is to have a positive outcome.

If the assessor feels that technological support, such as screen readers or voice-activated software, would be appropriate, then this should be made clear in the report. If the student is eligible for the DSA, a 'Needs Assessment' will be required in order to specify the technical support in more detail.

Study skills training may be beneficial and the assessor is in a good position to indicate where the focus should be placed; possible areas include memory or revision strategies, examination techniques, organisational skills, reading strategies, essay planning, learning medical/technical spellings, writing skills, word-finding strategies, or spoken presentation skills.

Recommendations for assessment adjustments should be made if appropriate. In many cases, it may be sufficient to recommend additional time for completion of written examinations. Some universities restrict the type of examination accommodations allowed, but they may include the use of word processors, amanuenses, or discretionary guidelines for the marking of coursework. Other arrangements may be flexible formats in coursework or examinations, the provision of questions on tape, or vivas and recorded submissions.

Other forms of institutional support, such as extended library loans, free photocopying, special small-group induction courses for the library or study skills workshops, may be available, and the student needs to be reminded of these at the time of the assessment and in the written report.

The thumbnail sketch of Ben (Figure 7.2) provides an example of how an assessment might benefit a student in Higher Education.

**Ben** (age 21 years)

| Standard Deviation | −3 | −2 | −1    0    +1 | +2 | +3 |
|---|---|---|---|---|---|
| Test | *Well Below* | *Below average* | ← *Average* → *range* | *Above average* | *Well Above* |
| Verbal ability | | | | | X |
| Non-verbal | | | X | | |
| SW reading – WRAT (untimed) | | | X | | |
| Sight words – TOWRE (timed) | | | X | | |
| Non words – TOWRE (timed) | | X | | | |
| Reading comprehension – Gray | | | | X | |
| Verbal memory – Digit Span | | X | | | |
| Spoonerisms | X | | | | |
| Spelling – WRAT | | | X | | |
| Copying speed – York Battery | | X | | | |
| Symbol Digit Modalities | | X | | | |
| CToPP Rapid Naming | | X | | | |

Ben is in his second year of a Social Policy with Social Psychology degree. He had learning support with English at Key Stages 2 & 3, but coped quite well with GCSE and A-levels. Since working at degree level, he has struggled with written assignments. He finds it difficult to plan and organise ideas in written assignments, which take him far longer than his fellow students to complete. He does not have his own computer but can use one in the university computer cluster when available. He also has problems taking notes in lectures and completing examinations.

His test results showed well above average verbal ability and good reading comprehension. However, significantly weaker single-word reading and spelling skills were revealed, especially under timed conditions, together with underlying weaknesses in phonological processing, verbal memory, rapid naming, writing and processing speed.

Ben has a dyslexic profile. His difficulties affect many study activities, but notably his ability to write in a fluent and ordered way.

*cont. overleaf*

Figure 7.2

The main recommendations to the university were:

Access to a word processor during examinations, since his handwriting deteriorates rapidly after a short period of time; additional time (25%) to complete each paper; departmental support – handouts in advance of lectures.

He was also advised to apply for DSA funding to buy his own computer and for specialist teaching in study skills, particularly the organisation of writing and use of *Inspiration* for mind-mapping on screen.

**Figure 7.2** (continued)

## Summary

This is an exciting and constructive time in HE, with institutions working to establish a culture of awareness and a framework of support. However, assessment at this level is no easy task, and assessors need to be conversant with the demands of HE, and with the subtleties and complexities of the issues involved. The life experiences the adult brings to the task, as well as the coping strategies they have developed over the years, combine to make their profile a rich and complex one. As assessors, we have to interpret the whole picture and create a positive way forward.

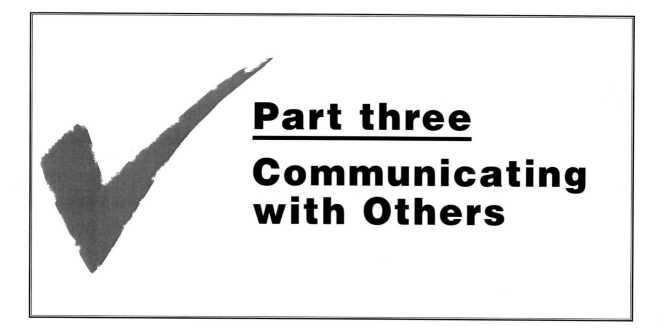

# Part three
# Communicating with Others

# 8 Planning a Teaching Programme

Sue Kime and Liz Waine

The summary to Chapter 1 gives six purposes for assessment, two of which are:

■ to recognise individual strengths and ways of working and to diagnose difficulties;

■ to plan intervention.

Both of these feed into the planning of a teaching programme. An appropriate assessment will have provided a list of strengths and difficulties and may have given some insight into the individual's learning style. However, one of the most difficult parts of writing a report is to translate these insights into a clear programme for someone else to follow. It is a time for clear thinking and one way to go about this is to ask yourself questions.

**What does the learner know?**

Look at:
- things he did well;
- strengths shown in assessment;
- knowledge which is already in place;
- developmental stage he is at.

**What does he need/want to know?**

Look at:
- breakdown points;
- areas where he lacked confidence and fluency;
- gaps in understanding/knowledge.

**What are the teaching implications?**

Think of:
- what needs to be taught;
- learning and teaching styles;
- modes of intervention (one-to-one, class, group).

**What are the priorities?**

Consider:
- long-term aims (the 'destination');
- short-term targets (the stops on the way to the destination);
- any urgent priorities (e.g. the need to build-in confidence and success before a challenge).

A good teaching programme will take all these things into account.

This section relates mainly to school-age learners, although some of the points are relevant to post-16 and adult learners. There are additional points relating to older learners at the end and in Chapter 7.

# Integrating into classroom practice and whole-school policies

6 *Specialised teaching strategies will be more successful, and of benefit to many pupils, if they are adapted for use within a class context, at the same time addressing the individual needs of specific pupils.* 9                                        (Howley and Kime 2003)

Whilst it is important to plan programmes for individuals, it is not likely to be possible to operate several very independent individualised programmes in the majority of classrooms. By integrating good practice into classrooms and whole-school policies, some learners will have all of their needs met. Others, who perhaps have more severe or complex difficulties, will have many of their needs met. This means any additional needs can be more easily addressed via group or one-to-one teaching.

Good classroom practice can provide multisensory teaching across the curriculum and make the use of practical resources routine across the age ranges, so that all learners are able to take advantage of such support when required. Individually planned programmes can then tap into these resources as necessary.

# Target setting

## Long-term aims

When planning a programme, the long-term aims should be identified first. These will link into National Curriculum levels and/or examination or vocational needs, as appropriate. It may be that more long-term aims are identified than can be realistically addressed at the time of writing the programme. However, it is important to identify all these aims because some may be partially addressed by good classroom practice and whole-school policy.

Once the long-term aims are established, the areas to be addressed by the teaching programme can be identified taking into account the learner's strengths and weaknesses, anything known about previous support and the educational setting. It is pointless to write a programme requiring an hour's one-to-one tuition a week if what is available is half an hour's group teaching and ten minutes one-to-one.

## Short-term targets

The next task is to set **Specific**, **Measurable**, **Achievable**, **Relevant** and **Time-related** (**SMART**) targets for each of the areas to be addressed:

**S**pecific: what will the learner be able to do by the end of the teaching programme? For example: Ann will spell *said, because, they, have* at word and sentence level.

**M**easurable: how will the learner demonstrate he/she can do what is required? For example: Ann will spell *said, because, they, have* with 100% accuracy at word level using an alphabet arc. She will spell them with 95% accuracy in dictated sentences during week 6 of this six-week programme.

**A**chievable: if the programme is planned for six weeks, will the learner be able to learn to spell the15 new words set as a target *and* meet the other targets in the programme? Would four new words be more realistically achievable? Does the learner have the relevant prior knowledge to achieve the target? Finding the right part of the dictionary quickly is only going to be achievable in a short space of time if the learner already has some knowledge of alphabet order. You should not be setting the learner up to fail.

**R**elevant: the target should fit into an overall structure which builds on previous knowledge. It should also be something which the learner *needs* and/or *wants* to learn. There is no point in teaching exam techniques to a learner who is not going to take exams. An older learner will not want to focus on basic spellings if his immediate need is for some subject-specific words he/she wants to be able to use at work. Motivation is a powerful tool in the teaching of learners of any age, but for older learners it is often the catalyst which enables them to succeed because, however difficult the task in front of them, the end result is either high on their list of priorities or it feeds an interest related to work or relaxation.

**T**ime-related: at what stage is the learner expected to demonstrate achievement of the target? If the programme is planned for six weeks, will achievement be demonstrated in the sixth week – or will that week be used for teaching, and achievement demonstrated the following week?

# Methods

Each short-term target should have an explanation of how the learner should work towards achieving it. What should the learner be doing in order to learn? This might, for example, include descriptions of the *look, say, cover, write, check* routine, the use of an alphabet arc for onset and rime activities, or the use of subject-specific words when working on syllable identification. The methods should be clear enough to enable the person teaching the programme to work effectively with the learner without the need for further explanation or research. The suggested methods should take account of the individual learner's interests and learning style wherever possible. The aim should be to use the learner's strengths whilst supporting his or her difficulties. Multisensory teaching methods are ideal for this. Using the learner's interests can make learning more pleasurable. When working on reading or study skills activities, the use of books and magazines linked to a hobby or interest will increase the learner's incentive to succeed.

# Resources

The resources required should be clearly stated and the list is likely to include many things readily available in the teaching establishment. If you think a resource may not be available – e.g. an alphabet arc in secondary school – it is worth providing information about a source. If you recommend a game, you might provide an example sheet produced on a computer (e.g. a set of cards for pelmanism using the words to be taught could be printed on a sheet of paper to be photocopied on to card and cut up for use).

Alongside this clear explanation of how to teach, you may well be able to identify published resources which could be used to achieve the targets – in which case you should provide a full reference for each of the resources you suggest. Published materials should not be used in place of setting SMART targets or providing information about how to teach. Telling someone to work through pages 3–8 of a scheme does not usually provide the impetus for exciting teaching. Nor is it a substitute for careful programme planning. In any case, the programme may not be suitable in its published form. It may need some adaptation for the individual concerned.

## *Pace*

The pace of the teaching is an important aspect. Individual parts of the target may need to be introduced over the period of the teaching, whilst previously taught information is practised and checked. Many published programmes introduce too many words or spelling patterns at once. The learner may need to focus on one new thing until it is secure before moving on. Your programme plan may indicate that one word or strategy is introduced in the first lesson and checked in the second lesson, and then the next on the list is introduced in the third lesson. The continued practice and checking of previous teaching should be built into the programme.

# Liaison

Liaison and review should be built into the programme plan. Where one-to-one or small-group teaching is required outside the normal teaching environment, it is important to provide information about liaison with other teachers. There is little point in working to build up a learner's confidence and self-esteem if attempts to use the new learning are not recognised and appreciated elsewhere in the establishment. Liaison with other teachers might be via a confidential sheet providing an overview of the learner's difficulties and how these affect his/her work in general, and suggestions of ways in which work might be differentiated by input or outcome (see Figure 8.1). Such a sheet would link easily into an establishment where whole-school policies and good classroom practice for supporting learning difficulties are in place, and it would be particularly important in establishments where this is not the case.

## *Links with home*

Where appropriate, consideration should be given to linking the teaching programme to available support at home. It may be appropriate to suggest games to support a spelling programme, possibly using computer software. Where support for reading is required games are often less threatening for the learner than reading to parents or carers. Often non-academic support, such as opportunities for sports, artistic or creative activities, is better because it builds up self-esteem and may provide an area in which to demonstrate a skill.

**CONFIDENTIAL**

**Information for teachers/tutors working with** [Name of student]

[Name of student] **has problems with:**

**It would be helpful if teachers/tutors would bear these factors in mind when working with this student:**

**Generally:**

**Where spelling is concerned:**

**Where reading is concerned:**

**When written work is required:**

**Please ask** [your name, tel, email address] **if you need any further help or advice.**

**Figure 8.1** Suggestions for Teachers sheet

# Review

The programme should state a date for review at the end of the teaching time, and it should be possible for this date to be brought forward if necessary. The review enables the learner's success in reaching the targets to be evaluated, and this evaluation will feed into the planning of the next set of short-term targets. The review should assess:

■ achievement of targets;

■ teaching methods;

■ teaching arrangements.

It is important to evaluate the effectiveness of the programme. You need to ensure that teaching is an efficient use of time and teaching resources, and that there is sufficient challenge for the learner to feel a sense of achievement. Individual or small-group teaching/learning time is a valuable resource which should be used to the best advantage for the learners concerned.

At this stage the long-term aims should also be reviewed so that appropriate areas can be identified for the next set of short-term targets. It may be that one area has received sufficient teaching input in the short term and it can be replaced with another for the next block of teaching.

# Older students

When writing reports on individuals who have left school, it is important to consider whether or not there is a need for a teaching programme. Some adults may have requested an assessment and report to provide themselves with answers about the root of their perceived difficulties and may have no desire to embark on a period of learning. However, individuals embarking on further or higher education may well want a programme which provides them with specific targets and teaching methods. Such a programme is more likely to focus on study skills, preparation for exams or on learning how to use hardware and software to support their studies. Some adults in the workplace may want specific teaching to overcome a difficulty at work – e.g. practice in taking down details of orders, or more general life skills (writing out a cheque in a shop used to be a common request but the use of technology makes this largely unnecessary now).

Targets chosen for any teaching programme need to be relevant to the learner and his situation, but this is even more important when writing programmes for adults. It may still be useful to write SMART targets but these will have a slightly different emphasis, as noted in the section on FE. Methods and resources must also be carefully considered and discussed with the learner. Many adults are willing to use multisensory techniques such as tracing spellings in the air and using tactile letters, provided the purpose and the rationale is explained to them. Resources must be age-appropriate: reading materials in particular need to be carefully chosen to be accessible and interesting.

Where teaching programmes are written for adults, the links to others should be carefully considered. In many cases adults will have the support of workplace, partners or relatives and suitable links should be discussed with the adult learner before being included in the programme. In some cases links may not be appropriate, particularly if the learner wishes to keep the learning support private. In this case the learner's wishes should be followed.

## Summary

- Teaching programmes should be closely linked to the findings of the diagnostic assessment.
- Where adults are concerned, the need for a teaching programme should be established.
- Long-term aims should link into National Curriculum, exam requirements, life skills or vocational needs, as appropriate.
- Short-term targets should be SMART.
- Methods of teaching towards the short-term targets should be clear.
- Liaison between specialist teacher/TA and class/subject teachers or college tutors, partners/relatives and the home/workplace (where appropriate) should be planned.
- Regular review should focus on the achievement of the learner and success of teaching methods, and results should feed into the new programme plan.

# 9 Working with Others

Jennifer Watson and Kath Morris

'Meeting the needs of children and young people with SEN successfully requires partnership between all those involved – LEAs, schools, parents, pupils, health and social services and other agencies. Partnerships can only work when there is a clear understanding of the respective aims, roles and responsibilities of the partners and the nature of their relationships, which in turn depends on clarity of information, good communication and transparent policies.'

(Special Educational Needs Code of Practice 2001)

This quotation highlights the emphasis now placed on a partnership approach to teaching and learning. Nowhere is this more important than in the interactions which take place in schools and colleges with regard to assessment.

This chapter will consider the place of teamwork and partnership in assessment, how to make it work, and who might be involved.

# Teamwork and partnership in schools and colleges

## Why is teamwork important?

The world of education was perhaps once a simpler place where all who took part 'knew their place' and were quite happy to let others get on within their individual areas of expertise. For example, in the 1970s and 1980s, a child in school with reading problems might be withdrawn from class and taught by the peripatetic remedial teacher. There was little communication between the visiting teacher and the class teacher beyond the occasional informal chat over lunch about how little Johnny was getting on. Unless parents were very persistent, they would often be left in the dark about the specialist help their child was receiving and how they could support it at home.

There was little or no attempt either to reinforce the specialist teaching in class or, on the other hand, to gear such teaching to classroom needs. We need to remember that some excellent work went on. However, it was often a 'one size fits all' sort of approach. This unfortunately often left the learner able to perform in his remedial lesson, but without making those vital connections to the day-to-day demands of the curriculum.

By contrast, we now live in the world of whole-school or whole-college approaches. In this climate of inclusion, class teachers, subject teachers and college lecturers are required to understand and respond to the needs of all members of their class. Specialist teachers are more likely to be guiding other professionals than teaching themselves; parents of school-age learners expect to be fully informed and involved in their child's progress; learners themselves are expected to be active partners in the learning process rather than passive recipients. Teamwork, partnership and good communications are essential requisites of this new environment.

# Effectiveness of teamwork

Whilst many would argue that individual teaching is still important for learners with dyslexia, this does not detract from the importance of a team approach. The whole is more than the sum of the parts, and the dyslexic learner is fortunate indeed if he works in an environment where both individual and in-class support is available as appropriate. The ideal world would be one where both he and his parents are involved in planning and reviewing progress, and where the whole school shares an understanding of both his difficulties and strengths. For all learners with difficulties, others' understanding of their needs is a powerful success factor.

# Good practice in teamwork

## Understanding roles

It seems a statement of the obvious to say that an understanding of the roles of others is important in building up teamwork. However, such understanding, though important, is merely the starting point. If working in an unfamiliar environment there is often a lot of work to be done in finding what local expertise is available, which links already exist and which need to be cultivated. For example, it might be important to find out which optometrist in the area has an understanding of dyslexia, or, within a school or college, what expertise there is among teachers and support staff. Some will have been on specialist training courses or will have experience within the family which has led to a special interest in dyslexia. They will be powerful allies within a school or college, or sometimes within a particular department.

## Important links in schools and colleges

If you are conducting an assessment outside your usual teaching environment, it is also important to know the organisational structure of the institution. As well as being in contact with class teacher and support assistants in primary school, it will very often be helpful to make links with head teachers, SENCOs (responsible for coordinating provision for children with special needs) and governors with responsibility for SEN. It is always an important courtesy to be seen and approved by the head teacher of a school where you are a visitor. In secondary schools the relevant year head may be more accessible than the principal and will have more knowledge of the learner you are assessing. The SENCO will be an important contact, as will both group tutors and subject teachers. In FE, Course Managers will know about the demands placed upon learners on their course and should coordinate information about any concerns from subject tutors. The Additional Learning Support Manager will have records of support given and will enable you to contact the support tutor working with your learner. The Examination Secretary in both schools and colleges will have a major role coordinating the assessment process, access arrangements and completing necessary documentation. However, all institutions differ in detail, and it is worthwhile doing a little research before conducting an assessment. In unfamiliar territory, it is useful to compile a personal pocket 'survival guide' of essential information.

## Patience, tact and diplomacy

Everyone likes his knowledge and experience to be appreciated, so that even busy fellow professionals are usually pleased to be asked for information and advice. On the other hand, they will like the demands on their time to be considered. Patience is needed if any lengthy contribution from them is required, such as filling in a questionnaire. Anything which will make the job easier will be appreciated; demands for time-consuming reports will not be well received.

Some, but of course not all, institutions are a minefield where undercurrents and rivalries can threaten good communications and therefore impact on a learner's wellbeing and progress. Tact and diplomacy is needed in navigating these troubled waters, as direct criticisms made by 'someone from outside' can often do more harm than good. In making decisions about intervention, the welfare of the learner involved must always be the prime factor. When suggesting a programme, if it is possible to recognise and build on what good practice already exists, this will be more productive than going in with no holds barred to suggest a complete turnaround of practice – particularly if you are a relatively inexperienced practitioner or new to the district!

Emails are wonderful but, especially in sensitive circumstances, they are no substitute for making personal contact.

## Ongoing interaction

The process of communication with others, which might be initiated through an assessment, is ongoing and dynamic. It is an important part of good practice to understand the processes involved in different sorts of assessment.

One example, which will be familiar to many readers, is the process of assessment for access arrangements in examinations. The decision as to whether access arrangements should be provided is not made on the basis of a one-off assessment but on evidence of a history of need. The evidence presented must take into account earlier assessments, usual ways of working, subject teachers' opinions as to the suitability of goals set, and the student's own preferences. Many people are involved in this process over a timescale which varies, but which could reflect the whole of a student's educational experience. Figure 9.1 represents the many people who will be involved.

Another example would be the route which might take a pupil in school through the stages of the provision made under the Code of Practice (2001). These stages include identification, School Action, School Action Plus, then – rarely in the case of a dyslexic pupil – an assessment for a statement of educational need. In

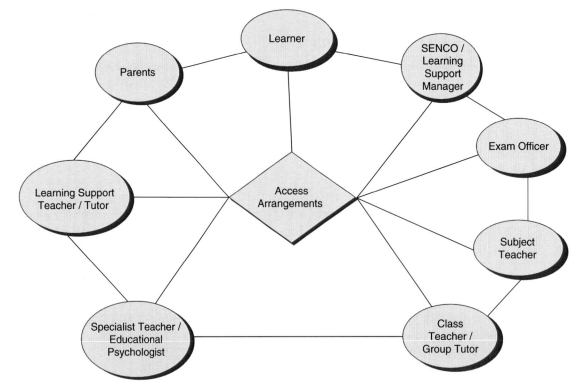

**Figure 9.1** Access arrangements – the people involved

this process, the learner himself, parents or carers, support assistants, class and/or subject teachers, the Special Needs Coordinator (SENCO) the head teacher, external support agencies, an educational psychologist and a speech and language therapist might all be involved at some stage.

Meticulous observation, record-keeping and review go with the teamwork needed to monitor and assess progress at each stage.

# Partnership with learners and parents – how to make it work

## Partnership with learners

6 *Children who are capable of forming views have a right to receive and make known information, to express an opinion and to have that opinion taken into account in any matters affecting them. The views of the child should be given due weight according to the age, maturity and capability of the child.* 9

(Articles 12 and 13 of the United Nations Convention on the Rights of the Child)

This statement appears up front in bold print in the Code of Practice (2001), but is still seemingly ignored in some assessment reports where programmes appear to be planned with no regard for the child's own aims, dreams, interests and obsessions. Even very young children can contribute ideas about what they enjoy in school and what they find difficult. No teaching programme will work without motivation. What better motivator could there be than a programme which, for example, draws on young Charlie's interest in dinosaurs or football – both great for teaching syllables and word building? Questionnaires for parents cannot take the place of establishing the sort of rapport which will make a young learner feel he is a partner in the assessment process, helping to find out things which will be useful for him. If he is feeling confident he is more likely to share information which might be useful – it could be something previously hidden, such as a bullying incident, or something very positive about how he managed to learn something really well the way Mrs Jones showed him the other day.

Older learners, after some initial reluctance, are often only too willing to share their experiences of life and learning in a confidential one-to-one interview. It is often the first time any one outside home has shown such an interest in how they, as individuals, cope on a day-to-day basis. Sometimes such histories can be very painful, especially for adults who have suffered a lifetime of humiliation because of their difficulties in literacy. As with younger learners, it is essential that careful observation of ways of working is part of the assessment, and that a programme of work is planned together, taking the learner towards his own personal goals and focusing on his interests and needs.

Partnership does not stop with the assessment. Reviews of progress for a learner of any age must involve him in assessing not only goals achieved and methods used, but also what worked best and what was not helpful.

# Partnership with parents

Those who are closest to the school-age learner with specific learning difficulties – his parents or carers – are those who may be most aware of associated difficulties. They may know that their child cannot remember that he went upstairs for clean socks or to wash his hands for lunch, that notes brought home from school are never delivered, or that he does not know which day of the week it is. They may not realise that these difficulties are aspects of dyslexia. A questionnaire used to investigate concerns (see page 183) can often provide reassurance for parents. Evidence (given with parental permission) from such a questionnaire can also be useful to supplement school records when assessment by another professional is requested.

While parents may remain anxious that their child is not acquiring literacy skills at the expected rate, their encouragement of their child is vital in maintaining his self-esteem. Encouragement of skills where the learner can show his individual abilities, such as swimming, rock climbing, art and design, can make a huge difference to confidence. In this context, also, it is vital that the learner's progress in literacy should be related to his own earlier attainment and targets and not constantly compared with his peers or siblings.

Parents can be advised of organisational strategies and routines to avoid panic and confusion – such as keeping timetables to show which days sports kit is needed or homework is due, checking the homework diary early in the evening, setting a time limit to homework in agreement with the school. These strategies also require commitment from teachers, checking that homework is given early in a lesson and that diary entries are correct, being willing to accept work produced in a given time, whilst acknowledging that it will not be as much as other pupils produce. However, such supportive liaison can be valuable in reducing stress on the dyslexic learner. Parents who are involved in supporting their child on a regular basis will make valuable contributions to review meetings and the continuous assessment of learner needs and progress. Where schools and parents work closely together it is more likely that a learner's needs will be identified as they occur. Close liaison can also enable the school to support parents, alleviating some anxiety and, hopefully, reducing any stress arising from the learner's difficulties.

# Working with those outside school – other professionals

With a deeper understanding of specific learning difficulties has come the recognition that there are links with other areas of expertise. Teamwork with other professionals can throw a new light on the problems experienced by an individual in school or college. Speech and language therapists, educational psychologists, occupational therapists and support teachers for behaviour and attention difficulties might all provide specialist support. Links with health services to promote a shared understanding of both health and educational difficulties are often important. Optometrists who specialise in visual problems relating to reading can also provide useful specialist support.

## *Speech and language therapists*

Where a learner has any difficulty with oral language, speech and language therapists (SLTs), with their detailed understanding of processes of speech and language development, can offer invaluable advice. Assessments are likely to include vocabulary, comprehension, use of grammatical rules, conversational skills, descriptive and explanatory ability, phonological and auditory processing skills. If the learner has been in school for some time, the assessment may also include reading and spelling. Analysis of results can have implications for planning the learning programme. In addition to work on a learner's articulation, phonological skills and basic language, speech and language therapists have expertise in identifying more subtle, higher-level language problems and can give advice on strategies to ameliorate these problems for learners.

## *Educational psychologists*

Work with an educational psychologist in assessment of a learner with specific learning difficulties can have any of four main emphases:

■ initial assessment of SpLD and advice on teaching and learning strategies;

■ statutory assessment for a statement of special educational need;

■ assessment for access arrangements to examinations;

■ in HE, assessment for Disabled Students' Allowance (DSA).

Before he or she can start to assess a learner's specific difficulties, a psychologist will need evidence of work which has already been done with the learner, their current attainment and records of specific interventions such as IEPs, and notes from review meetings. In schools, the learner is likely to have spent some time at the SEN Code of Practice 'School Action' stage, with progress routinely monitored, and at 'School Action Plus' with additional support.

Educational psychologists have access to a range of tests and assessment materials that are 'closed' to teachers. Where an educational psychologist is involved in the assessment of SpLD, the pattern of results obtained in testing should inform subsequent advice on appropriate teaching and learning strategies.

If a statutory assessment for a statement of special educational need is to be carried out, the educational psychologist will prepare a detailed assessment of the learner's general abilities, current attainment and underlying sub-skills. This will be accompanied by reports from school and from other professionals involved with the learner. The teamwork involved in preparing a submission for a statement of special educational need may, indeed, be significant in ensuring provision for a learner. However, it must always be remembered that this is a dynamic process and further teamwork will be needed to update any assessments in order to ensure that provision remains appropriate.

## Occupational therapists

Many dyslexic learners are observed to have difficulties in fine motor skills (particularly handwriting, developmental coordination disorder (DCD) often referred to as 'developmental dyspraxia'. Dyspraxic difficulties may include poor muscle tone, clumsy/inflexible movement, unclear hand preference, avoidance of mid-line crossing, left–right confusion and bilateral integration problems (difficulty in coordinating both body sides). Where such problems are observed, learners might be referred to an occupational therapist (OT) for assessment. The OT can offer recommendations for direct therapy or school- or home-based programmes. Some schools have found it beneficial to organise small-group sessions, supervised by an appropriately trained support assistant, to implement the OT recommendations. Learners who experience difficulties in handwriting and spelling associated with dyspraxia may also benefit from the multisensory strategies used in teaching dyslexic learners.

## Support teachers for attention and/or behaviour problems

Just as some dyslexic pupils also show dyspraxic difficulties, some may have difficulties in attention and/or behavioural control. Behaviour support teachers are skilled in observing and assessing the needs of children who have an attention deficit and those who have behavioural difficulties. They can offer advice in classroom management strategies to help the learner remain on task, make practical suggestions to overcome the short-term memory problems associated with difficulties in paying attention, and (if necessary) suggest appropriate reward systems to encourage sustained concentration.

# Summary

- Teamwork in supporting learners with special educational needs is both important and effective.
- For good practice to be maintained, there is a need for:
  - development of links with key personnel within a school or college;
  - understanding of and respect for the roles of others involved;
  - patience, tact and diplomacy;
  - ongoing interaction between all involved.
- It is important that learners of all ages are considered as partners in the assessment process.
- Parents of school-age learners know more about their children than anyone and must be involved.
- Assessment and advice from other professionals can inform the assessment and planning of provision for pupils with SpLD.

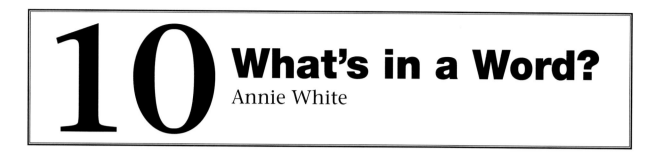

# 10 What's in a Word?
Annie White

'People may forget what you said and they may forget what you did, but they will never forget the way you made them feel.'

(Maya Angelou)

*'Sticks and stones may break my bones, but words will never hurt me'* is a familiar refrain from the playgrounds of our childhood – but, even as we chanted it in the faces of our tormentors, we knew, deep down, that it wasn't true. For words can wound, ill-considered sentences can sting and tactless text can cause severe bruising. These considerations should be borne in mind when writing diagnostic assessment reports.

In Chapter One we read that '. . . *purpose and intended audience will influence the way the . . . report is written . . .'*. In this chapter we will examine this statement in a little more detail – with regard to both the format of the report and the language that is used. We shall work through the various sections of a report (underlying ability, achievement, etc), discussing purpose and audience (and the effect both these will have on the language used) as we go.

# Background to assessment

This part of the report summarises the learner's previous history and experience. These are sensitive areas and the way they are approached can set the tone of the whole report. As in the rest of the report, be both clear and succinct. You may have collected a large amount of background information, but it is neither necessary nor desirable to include all of it. It is important to explain the purpose of the assessment and clearly identify at whose request it was carried out. In most cases, this will be a vigilant Special Needs/Learning Support Coordinator, working in a school or college. This is the most straightforward case, especially if the intended recipient is this same person.

However, this will not always be the case and, where parents have made the referral (usually because they are disappointed with the school's reaction to the problem), a little tact and diplomacy are required. In such cases, it is best to acknowledge that the child is happy enough in the present teaching environment. This is important if teachers and support assistants will be reading the report with a view to implementing any recommendations. Nothing will be gained by starting off the report with a statement like *His parents feel that Billy has been let down badly by the school and are desperate for advice*, even if this is closer to the truth.

Tact and diplomacy will also be required in those cases where this background information contains relevant information that is sensitive in nature. This might be the case if one of the parents is dyslexic or if there is a divorce pending. Permission must be sought from the parents before such information is presented to the world.

When writing assessment reports for adults, it is equally important to get the report off to a positive start and seek permission to include sensitive background information. Almost certainly, the adult subject of the assessment will be the first person to read the report – indeed, it is good practice to ensure that this always happens. The assessor and subject can then discuss any areas for concern before the report is passed on to a wider audience. In these cases, a useful way to explain the purpose of the assessment is *to gain a greater insight into his/her strengths and difficulties*. The psychological impact of reading the words *greater*, *insight* and *strengths* (all very positive concepts) before getting to the word *difficulties* (almost an afterthought) will put the reader in a positive frame of mind for what is to come. Once again, nothing is to be gained by plastering across this front page the fact that *Jenny is struggling to keep up with her coursework and her tutors despair of her*. Everyone may know that, but it is not the *purpose* of the assessment. The purpose is to try to find out *why* this is happening and try to work out some solutions to the problem.

# Underlying ability

The purpose of this section is to give the reader a broader perspective on the person who has been assessed. The school/college, the parents and even the subject himself are all only too aware that he has difficulties with spelling, reading or whatever. What they don't necessarily know is that he may well have potential in areas that are not readily identified in the current system of education. All parties concerned need to know what strengths he may possess (in contrast to the difficulties) and what the implications of the findings are.

As a starting point, it is helpful to explain the nature of the tests that have been used: to detail what was required of the subject during the assessment and to illustrate this with a few well-chosen examples. It cannot be assumed that the readers of these reports will be familiar with the finer points of Raven's Standard

Matrices (for example) so they will need to be talked through this. It is important to explain the tests in plain English: copying verbatim from the manual is not usually to be recommended. For example, introduce the Raven's Standard Progressive Matrices by saying this is a test of non-verbal reasoning ability and involves no words or reading. The testee is asked to choose a pattern which completes a sequence of given patterns.

# Non-verbal ability

The most important thing to remember in this section of the report is that conclusions regarding 'intelligence' cannot be drawn from the tests of non-verbal skills that are available to specialist teachers. Good non-verbal ability is usually taken as an indicator of aptitude for learning through direct experience, using logic and reasoning. This is only one small facet of intelligence.

The second most important consideration is the reporting of the scores. For a really high score, the phrase *excellent logical reasoning skills* could be used. For many dyslexics, this will be the first time that they have been described as being *excellent* at anything and it could make a good positive start to the report. The same will be true if these same skills are found to be *good* or even *at the expected standard for this age*.

Clearly, there will be instances where these scores fall *below* the expected standard. In these cases how much kinder to say this (especially if the scores fall just below the lower limit of the average band) than to use words such as *poor* or the dreadful *intellectually impaired* from the Raven's manual. Younger children (up to about eight years) with low scores could be described as *less well developed than is usual for his age*, as there is a possibility that they may catch up.

As there is a veritable minefield out there when it comes to reporting findings in a qualitative way (as opposed to the *quantitative* standardised scores and percentiles), the model of the normal curve of distribution (see Chapter 11) may prove helpful. Following this model will help to avoid the pitfalls that can sometimes occur when following test manuals to the letter. For example, a Raven's score at the 75th percentile is described in the manual as *above average*. When this same score is converted to a standardised score (of 110) it becomes *a good average*. Assessors who are relatively new to the practice tend to copy verbatim from the different manuals and this can have the effect of confusing the reader.

Still on the subject of consistent scoring, it is recommended good practice to present all scores as standardised scores rather than as a mixture of standardised scores and percentiles. Most of the assessment manuals now have a section where these transcriptions are made: even if the test manual that produces a score as a percentile (e.g. Raven's Matrices) does not have such a chart, other manuals will have (e.g. WRAT–3). Consistency is not the only issue here. If low scores are being reported, it is much less disturbing (either for the parent or the subject himself) to read about *a slightly below average score of 84* (standardised score) than *a below average score at the 14th percentile*. Psychologically, the former seems far more acceptable.

# Verbal ability

The same caveats apply to making assumptions about 'intelligence' based on scores of verbal ability as to making assumptions based on non-verbal ability. Knowledge of vocabulary is just one aspect of language development – and in turn, just one facet of intelligence. Granted, it is likely that a student who has excellent levels of receptive vocabulary (as measured by a test such as BPVS) will be able to cope with the language of the classroom better than the student whose lexicon is comparatively weak.

However, it is not a foregone conclusion that he should *do well in his studies*. The situation will be more complex than this: the student may well have great difficulty finding the correct spelling for all that vocabulary in his head and still not do himself justice in his written work.

When drawing conclusions from these results of verbal assessments, it is best to keep it simple and report a *good understanding of spoken vocabulary*. It is always good practice to include a couple of well-chosen examples of the level of vocabulary that was known. This is true regardless of the age of the subject. Seven year olds want others to know that they understand the meaning of *geriatric*; 47 year olds love to be reminded that they know the meaning of *terpsichorean* (especially if the assessor did not).

As with non-verbal skills, low scores need to be handled with tact and diplomacy and the word *poor* should be avoided at all costs. Sometimes the subject of the assessment may feel embarrassed by a lack of knowledge of vocabulary. This is particularly true of older secondary students and adults. If this is the case, they can sometimes be reassured that extensive vocabulary knowledge is acquired mostly via reading. Almost certainly, the person in question will have had difficulties with reading at an early stage of his life, even if they are reading at a functional level now, and this will have affected the desire to read and acquire new vocabulary. Ideally, this reassurance will have been given verbally at the assessment, and it could be helpful to include a reminder in the report.

# Attainments

It is a good idea to start this section with a discussion on spelling and writing: the implications relating to reading can be dealt with later. The reason for this is that there will be many, many cases where the level of written vocabulary falls far short of the level of receptive vocabulary detailed above, and this will be one of the most important points to be made in the whole report. Writing in this order will give the report a sense of continuity.

Almost certainly, the assessor and subject discussed any such discrepancy during the assessment process and it is a good idea to report any such conversations. This will have the effect of making the subject feel that they have been an important part of this assessment process (which, of course, they have).

When analysing the results of any assessments of literacy (reading or spelling/writing), be particularly mindful of the sensitivities of your readers – particularly if they are older secondary students or adults. This is the area where they will feel most vulnerable. It may be just about acceptable to them to have difficulty completing strange diagrammatic puzzles or repeating strings of digits in reverse order. After all, other people might find these tasks tricky. For most of the older children and adults undergoing assessment, it is a great source of embarrassment to them that they cannot read and spell as well as their peers. This is often the part of the assessment that they dread most and this will be the part of the report they will be most nervous of reading.

It is far better to focus in a *positive* way on the *strategies* that have been used to decode/encode unknown words. For example, *Ben used context to self-correct the word 'conversion' (originally read as 'conversation')*. Or *Amy used her knowledge of phonemes and common suffixes to spell 'physician' ('fizition')*. Do not adopt the more negative approach of listing all the errors made (*so* demoralising!) and trying to categorise them. The former approach, apart from being more positive, is also more succinct, as just one or two errors can be produced to illustrate each observed strategy. As if all that weren't enough, it will also prove helpful when writing the teaching programme, where the emphasis will be on teaching those *strategies* that are not being used effectively. Obviously, the errors will need to be examined in detail to inform the setting of SMART targets for reading and spelling in the teaching programme, but they do not need to be listed in their entirety in the main body of the report.

# Further diagnostic assessment

When describing tests of phonological awareness and memory, the language used must be succinct and crystal clear. Most people are aware of what is involved in spelling and reading tests. Few will have encountered these more specialist areas. Think through what the test really asks of the learner and use language which is accessible rather than quoting technical jargon from the manual. Specific examples of test items usually aid clarification.

Again, when reporting the findings, do so sensitively – particularly where the scores are below the expected standard for the age group.

# Additional guidelines as to the wording of reports

The whole report must be written in the third person: *The following tests were administered* sounds so much more professional than *I asked Jack if he would do the Digit Span next.* Similarly, when making mainstream teaching recommendations, it is better to write *It is common practice for subject staff to provide technical vocabulary at the start of each term* than to write, *in my school, subject teachers . . . .*

As a general rule, a firm conclusion relating to whether or not the subject is dyslexic is not expected. Primarily, the report should provide an individual profile of strengths and weaknesses with a view to informing good teaching practice. However, there will be instances where a label is sought, along with the reassurance that the label brings. This is particularly true of the adult dyslexic, who may well have spent many years pondering over the exact nature of the difficulties he is faced with. There will also be many parents who need to be reassured that their child's difficulty is recognised and that it does have a name.

Sometimes the scores may not correlate with the assessor's (or a parent's/class teacher's) intuitive perception of the subject's true capabilities. This is particularly true where the subject is reluctant to take risks and requests that the subtests be terminated as soon as he is less than one hundred per cent certain of the answer. This is more likely to happen in tests of underlying ability than in the tests of achievement – possibly because the nature of these assessments is foreign to the subject and, consequently, he feels more vulnerable. In contrast, struggling to read and/or spell is an everyday occurrence, so he may be prepared to persist at these tasks for longer. This reluctance to take risks is a valuable indicator of a crippling lack of confidence and should be included in the report as relevant test behaviour. The reader should be encouraged to bear this in mind when interpreting the scores. The standardised scores only tell one small part of the story.

Hopefully, the assessment process will have generated valuable insights into the subject's perception of the difficulty. He may also have detailed coping strategies that he has developed. It is a good idea to weave these snippets of information into the fabric of the report – this will give it an individual touch. The exception to this rule would be if the subject had confided that he felt *stupid*. This word (or any other equally derogative term) should never appear in a report, even as a direct quotation. It is one thing for a vulnerable person to confess such a thing in the intimacy of the assessment room; it is quite another to have it in print for the whole world to read. An assessor is in a position of trust and should be ever mindful of the responsibility that this entails.

As noted at the beginning of this chapter: *'People may forget what you said and they may forget what you did, but they will never forget the way you made them feel.'*

## Summary

- The wording of the report is crucial.
- It is important to administer and score the tests correctly. It is important to interpret those scores correctly when making comparisons both to the population as a whole and to the patterns associated with specific learning difficulties.
- All this pales into insignificance compared to the power to enhance or damage someone's self-confidence and self-esteem, depending upon the words chosen to express these interpretations.

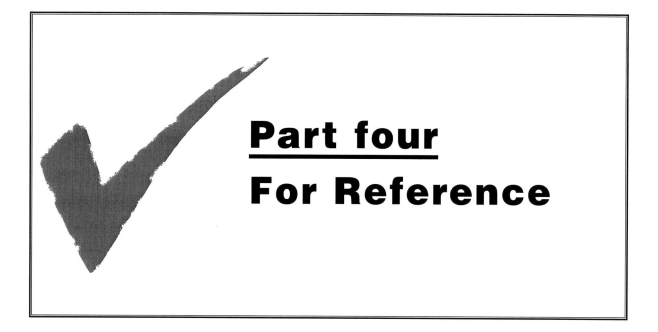

# Part four
# For Reference

# 11 Basic Concepts in Psychometrics
## Gill Backhouse

In this section, you will find a brief summary of some of the most important issues you must understand when choosing, using, scoring and interpreting the results of standardised tests in an educational setting.

There are two main types of standardised test:

1 *maximum* performance – where the testee has to do the best he can, as in single-word reading tests;

2 *typical* performance tests – which assess how the testee generally behaves, thinks, feels, etc, such as questionnaires.

For assessment of learning difficulties, tests of maximum performance are usually used.

# Choosing standardised tests

Test manuals vary regarding the amount of technical information they give. The contents range from basic facts to a large amount of complex statistical information, generated during the test development and standardisation. The amount of work involved in gathering this data is very considerable and is the reason why tests are expensive. You should be wary of tests developed by individuals or small organisations that may not have the financial resources or expertise to support the proper development of tests.

## The standardisation sample

Every time we look up an individual's test results in norm tables, we are in effect comparing his performance with that of the group used during the test development and standardisation. The larger that group, and more widely distributed across different areas (inner city, suburban, rural, etc), the more likely it is that the statistics regarding what is average, above and below, are meaningful and 'true' for the population as a whole.

For example, a reading test developed and standardised in grammar schools in one of the counties that still retains the 11+ will probably produce a different value for 'average' from one developed in non-selective schools in one of our more deprived inner cities.

Furthermore, since language, literacy standards and other attributes within both school and general population are constantly evolving, norms established several decades ago may not be fair representations of the population now.

The use of *equating* techniques, where testees take a new test and a recognised standardised one, is a powerful method of linking or equating standards and gaining reliable information using smaller samples of students.

**Action:**

Choose tests which have been recently standardised on, or equated to, a large, nationally representative sample.

The **age-range** of the standardisation sample is also extremely important – particularly during the primary school age when development of skills and knowledge is much faster than later on. This is why some tests provide separate norm tables for each six months during the early school years, then expand the age groups to one year in the secondary phase; as abilities 'plateau' in adulthood, they are given 5- or 10-year bands thereafter. Norms for 7 year olds will not be appropriate for most 6 or 8 year olds, but those for 16 year olds may not be too far from the mark for 25 year olds (but see page 159 about age-equivalent scores).

For statistical reasons, tests do not discriminate well at the extremes of their age range, and so best practice is to use tests for individuals whose ages are well within the test 'ceiling' and 'floor'.

**Action:**

Choose a test which more than covers the age range of the students you are assessing.

## *Reliability*

The reliability of a test reflects the extent to which it consistently measures the target skill(s). There are many ways of assessing reliability, each with its own advantages, and so reliability is not a fixed quantity. You will find details of the methods used in the test manual. Important aspects are:

**Test-re-test reliability:** testees should obtain the same scores if they take the test on 2 separate occasions. This is an important issue where there are parallel forms.

*Note:* In the assessment context, retesting within a short period of time is likely to produce a higher result due to learning that occurred during the first trial and so is not recommended. (During the standardisation process this is accounted for.)

**Administrator/interscorer reliability:** the same results should be obtained no matter who is administering or marking the test.

Data about the **internal reliability** of a test is usually represented by reliability coefficients. The **reliability coefficient ($r$)** indicates what proportion of the test variance is due to 'real' individual differences – for example, if $r = 0.87$, that means 87% of the variance is 'true' and 13% is likely to be due to sampling error. The higher the reliability coefficient of a test (up to 1.0 = perfect reliability), the more confidence may be placed in the consistency and precision of the results it generates. Look for values above 0.8 and preferably above 0.9. The lower the reliability, the less confidence you can have concerning the testee's real ability, based on that particular test result.

An often-quoted measure of internal reliability is known as Cronbach's alpha. This checks to see what proportion of the testees get questions of differing difficulty correct. For example, only the best should get the hardest ones correct. Values over 0.8 indicate well-designed and balanced tests that should enable differentiation to occur.

When all the items in a test are 'operating' (i.e. not too difficult or too easy) then the more items there are in a test, the greater its reliability. Therefore the results of short tests – in terms of number of items – should never be relied upon in a formal assessment, without a great deal of complementary and supporting evidence.

*Note:* A test such as the **Test of Word Reading Efficiency** (TOWRE) may be short in terms of time taken – because it is a speed test. However, the number of items to be read in 45 seconds is high, as are the reliability coefficients.

A number of computer based tests now screen individuals to ensure they only attempt questions of appropriate-level difficulty. This has the advantage of not wasting time and effort on too easy or too hard questions and still maintains reliability. The minimum number of items in a multiple-choice test should be 30, pitched at around the appropriate level.

**Action:**

Choose tests with high reliability coefficients and a goodly number of items to be tackled by the testee.

# Confidence bands and standard error of measurement

Some test manuals provide data regarding *standard errors of measurement* and *confidence bands/intervals* – either in the norm tables (e.g. **Neale Analysis of**

**Reading Ability**) or in the chapter about test reliability
(e.g. **Comprehensive Test of Phonological Processing**).

Standard errors of measurement (SEM) provide a 'ring of confidence' around a particular test score, since there is always the possibility of a discrepancy between a person's 'true' and obtained score. (Psychological testing is not an exact science!) The SEM is the likely size of this discrepancy, and confidence intervals are based on SEMs. They are usually defined thus:

- it is 68% certain that a person's 'true' score will be within the band of scores lying 1 SEM either side of his obtained score;

- it is 95% certain that it will be within plus/minus 2 SEMs of his obtained score;

- it is 99% certain for the range 3 SEMs either side.

There is an inverse relationship between the reliability coefficient of a test and its SEM. A highly reliable test will have a small SEM and so each obtained score is likely to be close to the hypothetically 'true' one.

# Validity

Validity studies tell you to what extent the test measures what it says it does: this has to be considered in the context of what the test user needs to know. Again, there are different ways of measuring validity because there are different aspects. The main ones are:

**Concurrent validity** shows that people who are known to differ on the task being measured, obtain correspondingly low, average or high scores on the test.

> e.g. Do good and bad clerks score well and poorly on clerical aptitude tests?

**Predictive validity** can be used to tell what will happen in the future.

> e.g. Do IQ tests predict exam grades?

**Content validity** relates to how well the test covers all relevant aspects of the skills being measured.

> e.g. Does an untimed single-word reading test measure 'real' reading ability: the capacity to read text with full comprehension straight away?

**Action:**

Choose a test which focuses on and measures the precise skills you wish to investigate. Select tests that provide sound evidence of their validity for the purpose.

Much information regarding validity (as well as reliability) is expressed in terms of correlations with results of other similar tests, exam results, teachers' ratings, studies with special groups and so on.

# Correlation coefficients

Correlation coefficients express the relationship between two variables, but do *not* necessarily mean that one *causes* the other – although it may. For example, there is a very high correlation between children's reading ability and the size of their feet – they both increase with age (the underlying factor), but neither causes the other!

Coefficients vary between minus one (perfect negative correlation) through zero (absence of correlation) to plus one (perfect correlation). So when a coefficient is less than one, one measure is influenced by some factor *not* found in the other.

If you multiply the decimal by 10, then square the result, an estimated percentage is obtained of the proportion of the two measures that represent a common factor.

As an example, let us consider the relationship between reading ability and verbal IQ.

> The NARA II manual shows that the correlation between verbal ability (as measured by the British Ability Scales) and reading comprehension (as measured by the NARA) is 0.65. So we can say that 42% (6.5 × 6.5) of what is measured by the two tests is common, but a host of factors other than those measured by IQ tests (e.g. literacy, motivation, quality of teaching, etc) are also highly relevant. However, the same table shows the correlation between verbal ability and rate of reading is lower (0.47), which means that only 22% of these two indices represents a common factor.

Looking at these concepts in another way . . . if everyone who passes test $X$ always passes test $Y$, then they are a perfectly correlated pair (i.e. the correlation coefficient is 1.0) and $X$ has a 100% accurate predictive validity for $Y$.

# Significance and probability

Against all this data about correlations – both in test manuals and research reports – you will find information about the significance of the results given as *probability* coefficients ($p$) or *significance*. These tell you about the likelihood of getting a particular result, or set of results, by chance. The smaller $p$ is (e.g. 0.05, 0.01, 0.001), the more significant the result: i.e. it would have been very unlikely to have occurred by chance.

# Using standardised tests

A principal characteristic of standardised tests is that the administration procedure, stimulus materials and scoring are prescribed and exactly the same for all who use and take them and match the method in which the test was standardised. Since all testees have (as near as possible) the same experience, differences in scores should reflect true differences in ability.

**Action:**

Make sure that you know and follow the procedures for administration of any test that you use. The manual will usually tell you the exact words to use and whether (for example) you may repeat a question.

# Understanding scores and interpretation of results

Most tests of ability and attainment, if administered to a large, representative sample of the population, produce roughly bell-shaped (normal) distributions, with lots of people scoring in the middle/average range (the 'central tendency') and far fewer having extreme (very high or very low) results.

The scales are usually converted so that every test has the same **normal probability curve** – a smooth symmetrical frequency curve having known mathematical properties.

**Raw scores** (direct numerical reports of performance, e.g. 60/100 on a test) are converted to **derived scores** – showing each person's relative position, compared to his peers, by using norm tables. There are three types of **derived scores**: Standard (or Standardised); Percentiles; and Age-Equivalent.

## Standard or standardised scores

These show the testee's position relative to the mean for his age group, using the **standard deviation** as the unit of measurement.

- The *mean* is the arithmetical average score for the reference group. (Other measures of 'central tendency' are the median and mode. The *median* is the middle score, and the *mode* is the most frequently occurring score in a particular set. These can be useful in situations where the distribution of scores is heavily skewed, or the mean is misleading because a few 'outlier' results are very different from the others.)

- The *standard deviation* (SD) is the average deviation from the mean – regardless of direction. Scores within 1 SD either side of the mean on any test are classified as 'average' (sometimes subdivided into 'lower' and 'higher').

If a **normal distribution** is 'sliced' into vertical bands 1 SD wide, a fixed percentage of cases **always** falls into each band and the overwhelming majority will fall within 3 SDs either side of the mean. The largest proportion of individual scores are 'bunched up' in the middle band (1 SD either side of the mean).

**Approximately two-thirds (68%) of individuals will fall in the 'average' range, defined in this way (34% either side of the mean)** – see Figure 11.1.

**Norms** tell you what the normal range of performance is, for a particular age range or group (e.g. 7 year olds, computer programmers, etc).

**Norm referenced testing** may be used for individual assessment (see **ipsative testing** below) or screening – to establish which members of a group (class) have abilities or attainments below a certain level, in order to trigger further assessment, learning support, etc, or special arrangements during examinations. The benchmark used for provision of learning support may vary between organisations such as schools and LEAs, according to their resources and may be, for instance, 2 or 2½ SDs below the mean.

■ **Standard scores are the most appropriate type of derived score to use when considering a testee's results**. They indicate how far away from the average level an individual is in terms of actual performance on a test. Furthermore, by measuring this distance in terms of standard deviation units, we can compare an individual's performance on one test with his results on another and derive a profile of strengths and weaknesses – as well as see how well he matches up to his peers.

## Percentile scores

These reflect the percentage of the group whose scores fall **below** that of the testee. A 10th percentile rank is therefore a low result (90% would do better) and a 90th (per)centile rank is pretty good as only 10% would exceed this score.

There is relatively *little difference* between the *raw* scores of a large *percentage* of individuals whose results are near the mean. Thus *percentile* scores between 17 and 83 are technically 'within the average range'.

**Percentile scores** magnify small differences near the mean which may not be significant; and reduce the apparent size of large differences near the tails of the curve: the difference, in terms of actual performance, between percentile ranks of 5 and 15 is far larger than that between percentile ranks of 40 and 50 (see example on page 157). Normalised **standard scores** avoid this, since the intervals on a standardised scale are all equal – but they are not generally well-understood by non-specialists!

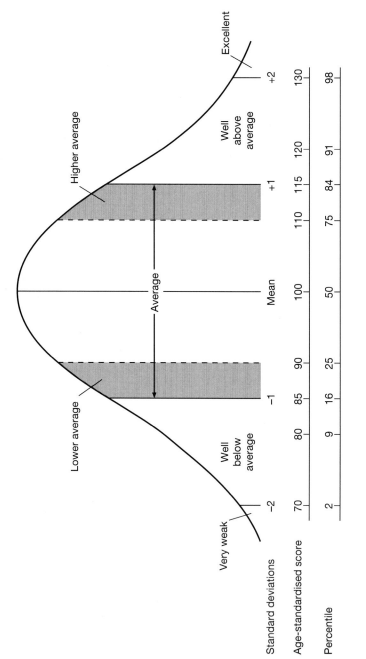

**Figure 11.1** The normal distribution curve, standard deviations, standardised scores and percentiles (from the Manual of the *Diagnostic Reading Analysis*)

## Hypothetical example

Say we measured 1000 adult women and found their average height to be 5 ft 5 inches.

How would we then define **below average** (short) and **above average** (tall), and how many women might be expected to fall into these categories?

This is where the standard deviation is useful since it is a measure of the **variance**, in relation to the **mean**, and is a generic mechanism for defining the above- and below-average 'benchmarks' on any standardised scale.

By finding the deviation (difference) from the mean of all 1000 women:

(e.g. if height   = 5 ft. 2 ins then deviation from mean   = 3 ins
..  ..        = 5 ft. 7 ins      ..     ..     ..   = 2 ins
..  ..        = 5 ft. 5 ins      ..     ..     ..   = 0 ins
etc.)

the **standard deviation** can be calculated by applying a set formula to the results obtained from the sample. Let us suppose the SD turned out to be 2 inches.

We can now define (statistically) the average range as between 5 ft 3 ins and 5 ft 7 ins and expect roughly 680 out of every 1000 women (68%) to fall between these limits. We can also define what we mean by *above* and *below* average in terms of height and, using the SD (of 2 ins), can predict that only 20 women are likely to be under 5 ft 1 in. and another 20 above 5 ft 9 ins (2 SDs above and below the mean) using our knowledge of percentiles.

| Mean | 5 ft 5 ins |
|---|---|
| **Standard deviation** | 2 ins |
| **Above average** (+1 SD) | 5 ft 7 ins and above (16% of popn) |
| **Below average** (−1 SD) | less than 5 ft 3 ins (16% of popn) |
| **Well above average** (+2 SDs) | 5 ft 9 ins and above (2% of popn) |
| **Well below average** (−2 SDs) | less than 5 ft 1 ins (2% of popn) |

As for percentiles, it is now relatively easy to see why they can be misleading. Out of our 680 average-height women, many are likely to be almost or exactly 5 ft 5 ins. It is clearly a nonsense to call someone who is 5 ft 4½ ins short, or another of 5 ft 5½ ins tall. You would be hard pressed to notice the difference between them and might easily misjudge who was the taller, even though one might be at the 35th percentile (5 ft 4½ ins) and the other at the 65th (5 ft 5½ ins). This sounds like a huge difference – but in terms of 'raw scores' is in fact negligible in relation either to each other, or to the mean.

If, however, we think in terms of SD units (of 2 inches) we can say one is taller than the other if there is at least 2 inches between them; or one is below average if she is under 5 ft 3 inches.

## The language used to describe scores

Different test publishers use a variety of verbal labels such as 'low average', 'superior' and so forth to describe different sections of the normal curve, which can be confusing. By far the safest and most meaningful thing to do is to stick to the correct statistical divisions based on standard deviations.

## The difference between 'below average' and a 'deficit'

Would it be reasonable to say that women measuring 5 ft 3 ins have a problem? Clearly not! However, being 5 ft 2 ins (1.5 SDs below the mean – in the **'moderate deficit'** range), may begin to affect life on the odd occasion. One's vision is restricted in crowds, choice of some clothes restricted to those available in 'Petite sizes' and it's hard to reach things off higher shelves – nothing serious, but a nuisance at times. At 2 SDs or more below the mean (**severe deficit**) – 5 ft 1 in. and below in this hypothetical example – more everyday things may become difficult: standard kitchen equipment is uncomfortably high and some careers, where there are minimum height requirements, are barred.

It remains to be said that 'deficits' are defined in relation to the demands made on the ability/characteristic measured. Height, for example, is only an issue in certain situations.

So long as we know the **mean** and **standard deviation** of any **standardised scale**, we can interpret a student's performance in relation to others in his age group, and also to his own score on other standardised tests. For both purposes, it will lead to sounder conclusions if standard deviation units rather than percentile scores are used. Some common standard score systems are given in the table below, but in the UK most tests now report a derived score using a mean of 100 and standard deviation of 15, and this is often called a *quotient*:

|  | Mean | Standard Deviation |
|---|---|---|
| Stanines (e.g. NARA, CAT[9] tests) | 5 | 2 |
| T-scores (e.g. BAS) | 50 | 10 |
| Deviation Quotients (e.g. WISC[10] IQ and Index scores; PhAB, BPVS) | 100 | 15 |
| Wechsler IQ and CToPP subtests | 10 | 3 |

---

[9] Cognitive Ability Tests.
[10] Wechsler Intelligence Scale for Children.

# Age-equivalent scores

The third type of derived score is the **Age-Equivalent** or **Test Age** (Reading Age, Spelling Age, etc). This tells you the chronological age, or age range, for which an individual's raw score is *average* or typical. However, **age-equivalents** become less and less appropriate as the age of the testee increases, since the rate of development of skills and attainments slows.

This is illustrated in the table below, concerning two pairs of learners.

A difference of one word read on the TOWRE (Sight Word Efficiency) by the two 7 year olds only alters the **age-equivalents** by 3 months. The Standard Scores are within the average range for both, and the **age-equivalents** reflect this.

Contrast this with the 24 year old reading just two fewer words than the 16 year old. The **age-equivalents** are roughly the same for both learners, but the 24 year old's looks horribly low: some 9 years below his chronological age. However, his Standard Score is actually within the average range for his age group (as it is for the younger student), because the norms at 16 are remarkably similar to those at 24. In fact the TOWRE 'collapses' the entire group between 17:0 and 24:11 years into a single table, whereas the 6 to 8 year olds (where development is very fast) have a different norm table for every six months.

| Chronological Age | Raw score | Standard score | Age-Equivalent |
|---|---|---|---|
| 7 yrs 0 mths | 31 | 98 | 7 yrs 3 mths |
| 7 yrs 6 mths | 30 | 91 | 7 yrs 0 mths |
| 16 yrs 6 mths | 92 | 98 | 16 yrs 0 mths |
| 24 yrs 6 mths | 90 | 91 | 15 yrs 6 mths |

A good rule of thumb is to avoid using **Test Age** scores altogether if possible, but especially for testees in the secondary and adult age range. If, for some reason, **age-equivalents** are required for someone in this older age group, you should take care to explain any large discrepancies between test age and chronological age.

Furthermore, you must **not** quote standardised scores if you have assessed a learner whose chronological age is higher than the test 'ceiling' (e.g. the BPVS with a 23 year old). In such cases you can only give qualitative descriptions of his performance in the report such as *well-developed*, etc.

# Ipsative testing

This term is used when a profile of individual strengths and weaknesses is based on a person's scores on different tests. Conclusions about his differential abilities, learning difficulties, attainments and so on are often drawn on the basis of contrasts of **one or more standard deviations** between standardised scores on different tests. It is generally acceptable to compare standard scores from different tests, provided the mean and standard deviation of both are known. For example, Ben's scores in CToPP and WRAT could be compared even though the respective tests used different scales (Figure 7.2, page 117). However, caution should be exercised if the two tests were standardised on very different populations or at different times (e.g. 1970 cf. 1990 – a generation apart).

Discrepancies in a learner's profile are a key factor in assessment, but we must be careful to distinguish between *deficit* and *discrepancy*. Few people perform at the same level in every test administered to them. One person may get well above-average marks on a verbal test and an average score for non-verbal reasoning. He is likely to find language-based subjects easier than practical ones. The difference of 2 SDs between scores is highly meaningful regarding his potential strengths and weaknesses. But since the lower score is not in the *deficit* range, it cannot be said that he has a learning difficulty! He may well have a problem, however, if he chooses to study technical subjects at A-level.

## 'Lower average' and 'higher average' scores

It is often the case that certain test scores are not quite in the *below average* range and yet all the evidence from the case history, our observations and other tests convinces us that there are sufficient grounds for diagnosing a learning difficulty. Given the degree of error inherent in tests it is sometimes justifiable to base conclusions on scores falling within the narrow 'slice', just within the outer edges of the average range, called **lower average** and **higher average**, as shown in Figure 11.1.

## Summary

- The first part of this chapter covered the essential knowledge required when selecting resources for particular assessment purposes. The second part provided the information needed when using, scoring and interpreting results properly.
- Significant **discrepancies** between a learner's scores on different standardised tests contribute to an understanding of his individual strengths and weaknesses. Significant **deficits** in relation to the national norms for his age will often help to explain difficulties at school or college.
- Evidence of deficits from standardised tests may be required before a formal diagnosis of a 'learning difficulty or disability' is accepted in some contexts, such as provision of LEA-funded learning support or 'access arrangements' during public examinations. A clear understanding of the basics of psychometrics is essential to interpret findings correctly and relate them to a particular context.

# 12 The Legal Framework

Nick Peacey

Article 2 of the First Protocol: 'No person shall be denied the right to education.'

Article 14 of Schedule 1: 'The enjoyment of the rights and freedoms set forth in this Convention shall be secured without discrimination on any ground.'

(The European Convention on Human Rights incorporated into English law in the Human Rights Act 1998)

This chapter examines the legal framework for the assessment of special educational needs and disabilities, particularly in relation to dyslexia.

# Defining assessment

We can separate definitions of assessment into three broad categories. The term can refer to:

- examinations and tests set to check progress at the end of a course or phase of learning;

- an exploration of the needs of an individual in relation to special educational needs or disability, access arrangements for examinations or any concern which may require intervention to minimise barriers to learning;

- the day-to-day checking of understanding in class and lecture room, sometimes known as *assessment for learning* or *formative* assessment.

The statutory frameworks now in place cover all three types of assessment. This chapter particularly relates to the second of the two categories.

# The scope of legislation and regulation

1   Much of the legal framework relates, with modifications, to the whole of the United Kingdom. It will be made clear if this is not the case. But this chapter

focuses on the English position: if you are working in Northern Ireland, Scotland or Wales, you should check details with the appropriate authority: Awdurdod Cymwysterau, Cwricwlwm ac Asesu Cymru/Qualifications, Curriculum and Assessment Authority for Wales (ACCAC), the Scottish Qualifications Authority (SQA), or the Northern Ireland Council for the Curriculum, Examinations and Assessment (NICCEA).

2  The core legislation relates to the following educational phases:

■ **Schools**
This area is legislatively the most complicated. The Education Reform Act 1988 set out the significant framework, by establishing the requirement for a National Curriculum, the pattern of Key Stages, and tests and tasks – National Curriculum Tests (NCTs, formerly known as SATs) for England and Wales. The Welsh Assembly has moved away from the NCTs model since it was established and the English system is now following suit.

■ **Further Education**
The Learning and Skills Council is the governing agency for all further education provision. The Learning and Skills Act 2000 set out its role and way of working in some detail, including sections on equal opportunities and assessment of learning disabilities. The Act covers England and Wales.

■ **Higher Education**
The foundation of all regulation for higher education in the UK is the Teaching and Higher Education Act 1998. This area includes the most independent institutions in the education system and so the Act is in a rather different style from that of the other two phases.

# Inclusion and assessment

The move towards 'inclusion' of learners with Special Educational Needs (SEN)/disabilities is influencing every type of assessment at every phase of education. *Inclusion* is often seen as simply synonymous with 'mainstreaming': moving those with SEN from special provision into mainstream institutions. But the broader meaning of the term, the process of allowing those from every minority to be valued and appropriately assessed and taught wherever they are learning, has gained great significance in recent years. Inclusion is increasingly backed by statute and legislation across the UK.

If we want a clear description of the principles of inclusive educational practice we need look no further than the Inclusion Statement of the National Curriculum (DfEE/QCA 1999a,b), which has statutory force in

English schools and is highly relevant to educational assessment everywhere at any age:

**A.   *Setting suitable learning challenges***

> *Teachers should aim to give every pupil the opportunity to experience success in learning and to achieve as high a standard as possible.*

**B.   *Responding to pupils' diverse learning needs***

> *Teachers should take specific action to respond to pupils' diverse needs by:*
> a)  *creating effective learning environments;*
> b)  *securing their motivation and concentration;*
> c)  *providing equality of opportunity through teaching approaches;*
> d)  *using appropriate assessment approaches.*

**C.   *Overcoming potential barriers to learning and assessment for individuals and groups of pupils.***

> ***Pupils with special educational needs***
>
> *Teachers must take account of these requirements and make provision, where necessary, to support individuals or groups of pupils to enable them to participate effectively in the curriculum and assessment activities. During end of key stage assessments, teachers should bear in mind that special arrangements are available to support individual pupils.*
>
> ***Pupils with disabilities***
>
> *Not all pupils with disabilities will necessarily have special educational needs. Teachers must take action, however, in their planning to ensure that these pupils are enabled to participate as fully and effectively as possible within the National Curriculum and the statutory assessment arrangements.*

There are clear messages here for those carrying out assessment:

**Section A** is about expectations. Assessors must be aware that an assessment which leaves a student feeling hopeless about any success, perhaps by failing to explore areas of strength as well as concerns, is not honouring the spirit of inclusion. Perhaps less obviously, considerable research evidence suggests that because of our capacity for imitation, removal from the company of those who are better at something than we are, whether for reading or anything else, removes role models and can depress expectations. Separation 'to sort out a problem' is not necessarily a good educational strategy.

**Section B** emphasises the need for every teacher at any level to plan and provide for diversity in a teaching group, as part of ordinary class preparation and the creation of a good learning environment.

**Section C** discusses specific planning and provision for individuals and groups.

The argument of these sections is that the better whole-group provision can be, the less need there is for specific arrangements for the needs of individuals and groups. So, for example, the better the quality of an examination generally, the less need there is likely to be for access arrangements for individual candidates.

Similarly, as activities considered special become standard, and as 'dyslexia-friendly' institutions become more and more established, the range of 'specialist assessment' required will change. Teachers and lecturers will be able to carry out straightforward assessments as part of their ordinary practice.

# The Disability Discrimination Act 1995 (revised 2001)

The Disability Discrimination Act (DDA) will increasingly affect assessment practice.

The original DDA gave extended rights to disabled people across the UK. But it did not fully cover education. (Some parts of the system were within its scope. For example, DDA Part 2, the employment section, has encompassed professional bodies' examinations – and hence the access arrangements for some candidates – since 1995.)

The Special Educational Needs and Disability Act 2001 (SENDA) 'enabled' the creation of Part 4 of the DDA, the education section. Now, across all phases of education, those responsible for provision must make 'reasonable adjustments' to avoid discrimination against disabled students.

The DDA Part 4 covers:

- existing and prospective students (so, for example, it includes enquiries and recruitment procedures for assessments and examinations, as well as assessments for entry to any sort of provision);

- private and maintained provision of whatever size;

- provision in post-16 institutions and provision for those under 16.

There are situations in which making an adjustment will not be 'reasonable'. The most important for the purposes of this chapter is that an adjustment must not undermine or lessen academic standards. So, if giving special treatment to a disabled student in the admissions procedure for a course will prejudice the standards by which every other candidate is selected, it is unlikely to be justifiable under the terms of the DDA.

As the SEN Code of Practice (DfES 2001: see below) does not apply to 'post-16 provision', the anti-discrimination duties on schools and local education authorities (LEAs) are significantly different from those on colleges and universities. For example, LEAs and schools must have strategies and plans which show how, over time, they will improve accessibility to the curriculum (which includes assessment of all types), the physical environment and written information for disabled students. Separate disability codes of practice are available for each age group (DRC 2002a, DRC 2002b).

*Note:* Some of the DDA's implications for Scotland and Wales can be explored by looking at Disability Scotland and Disability Wales/Cymru pages on the website of the Disability Rights Commission (DRC 2004).

# The SEN Code of Practice (SEN Code) (revised 2001)

The SEN Code of Practice only applies to the education of children and young people with SEN in schools. The first version, published in 1994, focused on the identification and assessment of special educational needs. The essential model was 'assess and provide for the individual', normally mediated through an individual education plan, with or without a statement of special educational needs.

The revised SEN Code assumes that teachers will normally plan for a diversity of learners in any class. So the goal of assessments is to decide on the 'additional or different' elements needed to support an individual's learning. The 'graduated approach' to assessment has three stages: School Action, School Action Plus (assumed to involve specialist advice with provision made by the school) and the Statement of SEN which normally involves additional resources provided in some way by the local education authority.

A key principle of the revised Code is that the identification of need is only useful if it improves the learning chances of the student, in class, gymnasium or elsewhere. Assessments which take place in isolation (those, for example, that do not involve any sort of liaison with the pupil's teachers or observation of the student at work without good cause) have become less prevalent for this reason.

The Code has its foundation in law in the Education Act 1996. Strictly speaking, schools are only required to 'have regard' in relation to the two earlier stages of assessment (i.e. can choose what they do, once they are clear what the Code suggests). The sections on the Statement, because of its power and enforceable access to resources, have the force of law.

# Precedent and the High Court

However, a straightforward reading of the SEN Code will not give you the whole story. Cases brought by those unhappy with decisions made under any area of the Code may go right through to the High Court. Once there, the High Court's decisions have statutory force. So, in relation to all the legislation described in this chapter, it is important to maintain a watch on the developing situation through websites, publications and Patoss or other voluntary or professional body membership.

# Assessment under the Learning and Skills Act 2000

The Learning and Skills Council 'must have regard' to the needs of persons with learning difficulties. The statutory basis for assessment is provided by Section 140 of the Act. This Act is striking throughout for the emphasis it gives to the Secretary of State for Education and Skills' direct responsibility for provision (elsewhere the responsibility rests on LEAs or institutions and the Secretary of State's role is to make sure the system works).

Section 140 seeks to smooth transition by an emphasis on assessment for those with learning difficulties who have a statement of SEN at school. It continues:

> *The Secretary of State may at any time arrange for an assessment to be conducted of a person . . .*
> *(a) who is in his last year of compulsory schooling or who is over compulsory school age but has not attained the age of 25,*
> *(b) who appears to the Secretary of State to have a learning difficulty (within the meaning of Section 13), and*
> *(c) who is receiving, or in the Secretary of State's opinion is likely to receive, post-16 education or training (within the meaning of Part I of this Act) or higher education (within the meaning of the Education Reform Act 1988).*

# The Disabled Students' Allowance (DSA)

Students in higher education are eligible for the Disabled Students' Allowance (DSA). This is a non-means-tested grant, payable to students, from their local education authorities. A needs assessment is normally required (see Chapter 7). The DSA covers three areas of support:

- general allowance – to cover, for example, insurance, computer printer ink;

- non-medical helper allowance – for example, note-takers, interpreters; purchase of appropriate support to develop study skills;

- equipment allowance – including assistive technologies such as speech output systems, speech recognition systems, alternative input devices.

# Assessment for access arrangements for examinations and tests

The Disability Rights Commission's (DRC) view of access arrangements was given by Gareth Foulkes at an ACCAC conference (Foulkes 2003).

*The purpose of an assessment is to determine the student's achievement or skills. Assessments must be rigorous regarding standards so that all students are genuinely tested against an academic benchmark. However, they must be flexible enough to allow all students an equal opportunity to demonstrate their achievement. In all cases, this means being very clear about what is being assessed so that modifications can be made without compromising standards – the aims should be to change the mode of assessment, not the way it is marked.*

## The national Key Stage test systems: the NCTs

Since 1988 formal testing systems of one sort or another have been in place across the United Kingdom for pupils at the ages of 7, 11 and 14. National government agencies monitor and regulate these tests. The Qualifications and Curriculum Authority (QCA) oversee this work in England. English and Welsh test systems have been very similar (though are now diverging), but differ substantially from those of Scotland and Northern Ireland.

## GCE, GNVQ, GCSE and VCE

The GCE A-level and GCSE examinations are the best known of a range of possible qualifications, including the GNVQ and the Vocational Certificate of Education (VCE) which are available across the United Kingdom. They have traditionally been taken by students aged 16 years or over. On 1 January 2004, the Joint Council for Qualifications (JCQ) took over representation of the major awarding bodies which serve England, Wales and Northern Ireland, including AQA, CCEA, City and Guilds, Edexcel, OCR and WJEC. The awarding bodies are independent institutions, which are themselves regulated by national government agencies. JCQ publishes annual Regulations and Guidance on access arrangements (see www.jcq.org.uk).

# *Universities and independent accreditation granting institutions*

As students move into courses of study designed for adults, they are likely to pursue accreditation approved by an independent institution such as a university or a professional body, such as the Chartered Institute of Public Finance and Accountancy, for example. The principles behind access arrangements remain the same in such cases, though the frameworks for regulation differ.

# *The two dimensions of a decision about access arrangements*

In granting any access arrangements we must consider:

- the assessment demands of the test or examination in question;
- the needs of the candidate in that assessment.

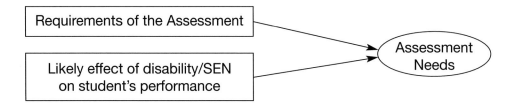

A study for the Schools Examinations and Assessment Council (1992) put it like this:

> *Special educational need should be considered in terms of its implications for assessment. It is necessary to show the **direct effects** of a precisely specified disability or learning difficulty **upon a pupil's performance in assessment situations**. . . . Special educational needs do not provide the most appropriate basis for determining **assessment needs**.*

So, for example, the QCA Key Stage Test Assessment and Reporting Arrangements normally allow electronic spell-checkers in any test except the spelling test. The assessment is testing the candidate's ability to spell, so, whatever the literacy difficulty, it would be inappropriate to allow the use of a spell-checker.

We should look for evidence of an individual's needs in relation to a specific assessment.

> *It is not the case, for example, that everyone with a "diagnosis" of dyslexia (or indeed with a statement of SEN) is automatically entitled to 25% extra time across the board – or that this is in their interests! The quality of their literacy skills may not*

*place them at any disadvantage in practical subjects, "multiple-choice" papers and so on. They may not know enough to be able to use extra time profitably – or "shoot themselves in the foot" during extra time by altering responses which were satisfactory.* ❜

(Backhouse 2000)

This is all, of course, equally true of students receiving the Disabled Students' Allowance for a university course. A 'diagnosed' label is needed for those resources to be provided, but that label cannot be the whole story on any support or access arrangements.

The shift from the assumption that a 'label' alone can identify special arrangements makes the involvement of teachers and lecturers in granting them highly appropriate, even if educational psychologists or others from outside the institution have a role.

❛ *It is sometimes the case, that candidates present assessment reports from independent practitioners stating that the student has a difficulty about which the school/college is unaware. . . . The guidelines for completion of both the Psychological and Specialist Teacher's Assessment Forms stress the importance of liaison between EPs/Specialist Teachers and centres in these matters. Liaison between assessor and SENCO is therefore necessary in order to meet the examinations boards' requirements.* ❜

(Backhouse 2000)

## 'Consistency' of access arrangements through educational phases

It is sometimes assumed that an individual should be granted identical access arrangements in a subject throughout their education. But, if the purpose of assessments differ, their access arrangements will need to vary. For example, there will never be complete 'consistency' between arrangements for the GCSE, GCE A-level, GNVQ and the Vocational Certificate (VCE) and the English Key Stage tests. The former offer employers and society a view of an individual's ability; the latter, while testing the attainment of individuals, are normally only a public resource for making judgements about institutional success.

# Bodies not covered by the revised DDA

It quickly became clear that regulatory authorities, such as QCA, and awarding bodies, such as Edexcel, were likely to be exempt from the DDA Part 4 (Education). Two developments since 2001 affect this position.

First, the DDA (Amendment) Regulations 2003 brought every professional or trade qualification which is *'needed for or facilitates engagement in a particular trade or profession'* within the DDA from October 2004. The DRC suggests that this will even include *'registration to practise in professions and trades, such as registering as a social worker, nurse or teacher; or as a CORGI gas fitter'*(DRC 2004).

Second, a further Disability Discrimination Bill is in draft. The Joint Committee of the Houses of Parliament considering the Draft Bill noted *'uncertainty about whether some standard-setting bodies, which set standards against which qualifications are awarded but do not themselves award qualifications, are covered by the Amendment Regulations'* and that *'the draft bill makes no specific changes to the current situation'*. The JCQ suggested that statutory control would reduce flexibility and increase bureaucracy without delivering benefits for disabled students. But the committee recommended that *'all examination bodies and standard-setting agencies are brought within the provisions of the DDA.'* The evidence of such witnesses as Gabrielle Preston, a parent of a child with dyspraxia, who *'stated that one examination body "refused to make any adjustments on the dubious grounds that they were not legally obliged to do so"'* (Joint Committee 2004), may have been persuasive.

# Looking ahead

## *The 'delegation' of resources*

The English government is encouraging a shift from the use of statements for the allocation of resources for SEN in schools. DfES-supported research argues:

6 *In recent years authorities with low levels of statements have increased SEN spending more than those with high levels of statements. Data from the case studies suggests that this reflects investment in building the capacity of schools to respond to wider range of pupil needs but findings are tentative due to the small sample size.*

6 *Key benefits of reducing reliance on statements include a fairer distribution of SEN resources, more support for more children and less paperwork and SEN-related bureaucracy. Elements that worked less well included continued variation in the capacity and commitment of local schools to meeting children's SEN across all areas and concerns about loss of "passported benefits" linked to statements.* 9

(Pinney 2004)

This move is challenged by many voluntary bodies. But the shift towards giving schools, particularly secondary schools, more control over funding decisions is unlikely to be reversed. This could help schools build accessibility into all assessment practice, but will undoubtedly increase demands for the accountability of individual institutions, their staff and those supporting them in assessments relating to SEN.

# Developments in the law

Overall, the law is likely to tighten its oversight of assessment practice and individuals will have increased opportunities to challenge institutions on discrimination in this area. The Professional Association of Teachers of Students with Specific Learning Difficulties (Patoss) now encourages any specialist teachers, not covered by institutional policies, to seek insurance against challenges about the consequences of their advice.

> *It is clear from the thrust of the recent opinions of The Lords of Appeal for Judgement in the Case of Phelps v. Mayor etc of The London Borough of Hillingdon[11] that Specialist Teachers (as well as EPs) have a duty of care to children with SENs with regard to the advice that they give. Therefore, they should ensure that they themselves are fully covered.*
>                                                                   (Backhouse 2000)

Schools and LEAs can build the improvement of equitable practice on assessment (through professional development, for example) into the Accessibility Plans and Strategies they must have under the planning duties of DDA Part 4. If they are systematically moving forward over time on this area, in partnership with stakeholders such as students and parents, they are in a strong position to meet individual challenges to their approach.

# The impact of the Green Paper 'Every Child Matters'

The Green Paper *Every Child Matters* (DfES 2004b), recently reinforced in the Government's ten-year SEN strategy *Removing Barriers to Achievement*, aims to bring resources and services for children closer together than ever before. The most powerful driver for this change is likely to be the planned single inspection regime, led by the Office for Standards in Education.

The implementation of the Green Paper will see '*a common assessment framework across services*' and the promotion of '*common use of language about SEN and disabilities.*' There is no place for assessment procedures which are not 'joined up' in the new framework.

---

[11] See House of Lords Judgements, Session 1999–2000; http://www.publications.parliament.uk/pa/ld199900/ldjudgmt/jd000727/phelp-1.htm

# 13 Resources

## 13.1 Miscue analysis  Gill Backhouse

Miscue analysis is a technique which enables you to assess the learner's strategies when he is reading continuous prose. It can be carried out as part of a prose-reading test or any suitably demanding text. Since about twenty errors are needed for the analysis, you need to have a good idea of his reading skills first, so that you can choose suitable material.

- If not using a test, photocopy the chosen text to use as a record sheet.

- Indicate *how* the learner attempts to read all the words with which he has difficulty. **Do not just put ticks and crosses.** Use a tape-recorder if you are inexperienced.

There are *two* stages in the analysis:

1  Catalogue all the errors made and consider the balance of error-types: for example, **Substitutions** (words read incorrectly, as other real words or as non-words) – 15: **Self-corrections** – 5: **Refusals** – 3: **Insertions and omissions** – 2.

*Note:* self-corrections are a good sign, as they show that sentence structure and meaning are being used to inform a second, successful attempt. If *said* is not recognised, is sounded out as 's – a – i – d' and then read correctly when its meaning had become clear, the reader is clearly beginning to use 'top-down' strategies.

2  Then, carry out the next level of analysis on just the **substitutions**. Draw up a table to show which cueing systems the reader has used for each one. Did he respond with a word that looked similar to the target (*grapho-phonic* cue)? Did his response sound OK within the sentence (*syntactic* cue)? Did his response make sense within the whole passage, showing he is making use of semantic cues and trying to read for meaning?

| *Target* and response | Grapho-phonic? | Syntactic? | Semantic? |
|---|---|---|---|
| *Certain* 'curtain' | - yes - | - no - | - no - |
| *Daring* 'darling' | - yes - | - no - | - no - |
| *Huge* 'large' | - perhaps (*-ge*) | - yes - | - yes - |
| *Concealed* 'hidden' | - no - | - yes - | - yes - |

Add up the number of positives in each column, and compare the totals. It becomes clear if the student is, for example, relying heavily on the grapho-phonic cueing system but not thinking about syntax, or making a real effort to gain or preserve meaning. 'Yes' in two (or all three) columns for the same word, would indicate that the learner is simultaneously processing at different levels – *word* and/or *sentence* and/or *text*.

This type of analysis will help you to decide on and justify your advice about how to help the poor reader develop more effective strategies.

# 13.2  Suggested format for diagnostic assessment reports

## *OCR report format*

This first example is suitable for many types of assessment report for which a set format is not specified. It is reproduced with permission from the *Tutor's Handbook, OCR Level 5 Certificate and Diploma in Assessing and Teaching Learners with Specific Learning Difficulties (Dyslexia),* copyright© OCR 2003.

### Section 1  Title page

| Teacher's details | name, qualifications and contact information |
|---|---|
| Learner's details | name, date of birth, address, school, college, chronological age, date of assessment<br>(identifying details should be removed where necessary)* |

* Please note that details identifying a learner should only be removed if the report is being submitted as part of an award.

### Section 2  Summary of standardised test results

| Underlying level of ability | full name of test (including edition number where appropriate); standardised score/percentile rank/age-equivalent category) |
|---|---|
| Attainments | |
| Further diagnostic tests | |

### Section 3  Analysis of learner

| Reasons for referral | |
|---|---|
| Background information | development and educational history; previous SEN identification and support; family history; relevant information from school/college/parents |
| Assessment procedure | including behavioural observations |
| Underlying level of intellectual ability | verbal/non-verbal tests; brief description of tests; reasons for administration; results and implications |

| Attainments | clear identification of strengths and weaknesses: sound-symbol correspondence; alphabet sequence<br>**reading** (single-word and continuous text); names of tests; results; analysis and comments on reading strategies (give two or three examples to illustrate your points)<br>**spelling** – single-word (title) results; analysis<br>**free writing** – comments on all relevant aspects (e.g. style, fluency, ideas, punctuation, grammar and syntax, handwriting, general presentation)<br>**other** – e.g. numeracy, tables |
|---|---|
| Further diagnostic testing and observation | reasons for choice of tests/procedures – e.g. phonological awareness/processing skills; auditory discrimination and short term memory; visual skills/problems; gross and fine motor skills |
| Conclusions | |
| Recommendations | |

## Section 4  Teaching programme

| Long term targets | |
|---|---|
| Specific targets for six weeks' work | must be SMART; should cover both basic skills and study skills; may include making use of appropriate aids and special arrangements |
| Suggested teaching methods/learning strategies/resources/pace | should be appropriate for a non-specialist teacher or learning support assistant to follow<br>ensure suggestions are not reliant on a specific published programme (it may not be available) |
| Suggestions for school/college support where appropriate | |
| Suggestions for parental support arrangements | e.g. reading or spelling games; supporting swimming or other opportunities for success |
| Review date | |

# Suggested format for DSA diagnostic assessment report

This second example is the proposed recommended format for assessments for Disabled Students' Allowance (DfES Working Party on Dyslexia 2004 – pro forma available from DfES website). They will be incorporated in the DfES guidelines for the assessment of SpLD in Higher Education (2005).

## Cover sheet

The candidate's name; date of assessment; date of birth; age at assessment; correspondence address; college/university attended; course of study (subject and degree); year and length of course (e.g. second year of four-year course).

Assessor's details and qualifications.

## Conclusion and summary

Diagnostic findings should be stated, with summary of evidence on which this is based; outline of effects of SpLD on student's literacy and study skills, taking account of compensatory strengths.

## Background information

Referral information; family, developmental and educational and language history; relevant medical information; summaries of previous assessment reports; student's perceptions of his/her difficulties and motivation for assessment.

## Test conditions

Brief statement about environment, comfort, interruptions, as well as health of student, attention, motivation, anxiety or anything else that might have affected results.

## Assessment

*(Reports of performance in individual tests should be prefaced by a brief statement about the cognitive function or attainment which the test is designed to examine, and a description of the requirements of the task for the student.)*

■ **Attainments in literacy**
**Reading:** single words (a graded, single-word reading test); non-word reading; text reading (both oral and silent); reading comprehension; qualitative analysis of errors, evidence of strategies such as whole-word recognition, decoding; fluency; reading speed (oral and silent) and ability to extract information from text; summary of student's reading profile.

**Spelling:** graded spelling test (single words); free writing; dictation of sentences (optional). Qualitative analysis of errors.

**Writing:** free writing analysed to cover vocabulary, ability to write grammatically, complexity of sentence structures, coherence of their writing; writing speed; and legibility of handwriting. Handwriting speed for copying should be reported separately.

### ■ General intellectual ability
Information about both verbal and non-verbal ability; observations about test performance; discussion of profile of scores, highlighting any significant discrepancies.

### ■ Cognitive processing
A range of tests selected by the assessor to probe relevant aspects of cognitive functioning: tests of working memory (if these have not been reported in the section under General Intellectual Ability); tests of phonological processing (phonological awareness and phonological processing speed); as relevant, tests of competence in numeracy and/or tests of motor control. Tests should be reported under separate headings.

### ■ Other relevant information
Use this section as appropriate to report on, for example, visual discomfort/Meares-Irlen Syndrome, signs of dyspraxia or ADHD.

### ■ Recommended support
Brief statement about the type of support that might help the student, particularly in relation to study-skills tuition; advice about the procedure for applying for the DSA.

### ■ Signed statement
Statement certifying assessment has been conducted and the report written in accordance with the DfES guidelines for the assessment of SpLDs in Higher Education (2005).

## Appendix
Tests used in assessment and summary of scores achieved.

# 13.3  Report checklist     Kath Morris

This checklist was originally developed as an informal marking aid for tutors. It can equally well be used for self-assessment.

## Background Information

| Good practice | Weak practice |
| --- | --- |
| Concise | Too long |
| Focused, relevant | Discursive |
| Objective | Anecdotal |
| Outlines learner's priorities for learning clearly | Disregards learner's priorities for learning |

## Choice of tests

| Good practice | Weak practice |
| --- | --- |
| Tests are age-appropriate, age of learner taken into account in number of tests used | Inappropriate for age and stage |
| Tests cover all important areas | Inadequate range of tests |
| Tests current | Out-of-date tests |
| Tests selected judiciously | Too many tests used, unnecessary repetition |
| Tests valid, well known and reputable | Validity of tests used questionable |

## Summary of scores

| Good practice | Weak practice |
| --- | --- |
| Scores summarised in clear table | Scores difficult to find, not summarised in tabular form |
| Correct transcriptions of scores | Transcription errors |
| Scores correctly calculated | Calculation errors |
| Descriptors of range used correctly and significance of these understood | Statistical concepts not understood (e.g. average range; below average, above average) |
| Test name given correctly, information given on edition used and test ceiling | Test names spelled wrongly or acronyms used without explanation |

## Interpretation of results

| Good practice | Weak practice |
| --- | --- |
| Discussion/interpretation groups tests logically (e.g. underlying ability, attainment, diagnostic tests) | Discussion/interpretation of results is muddled and illogical. |
| Relevant links between results are recognised and discussed | No links are made between different test results |
| Observations of learner's strategies and learning style are discussed with insight, citing appropriate examples | Discussion does not take into account observations of learning style and strategies |
| Report clearly interprets information in relation to norms | Norms do not seem to be understood – e.g. where reading age matches chronological age, this is not recognised |
| Where inferences are made they are treated cautiously and presented as suggestions rather than facts | Incorrect or unreliable inferences are made – for example in relation to intelligence – and treated as fact |
| Interpretation recognises strengths as well as difficulties | Interpretation is unduly negative |

| Good practice | Weak practice |
|---|---|
| Phonological awareness and its importance as a skill underlying literacy clearly understood | Phonics confused with phonological awareness |
| Strengths and difficulties summarised clearly | Strengths and difficulties not summarised |
| Detailed interpretation of what is known and where breakdown points occur | Vague: gaps in knowledge are not defined – so report gives no specific information on which to base a programme |

## Recommendations and teaching programme

| Good practice | Weak practice |
|---|---|
| Recommendations/programme show clear links to the individual pattern of strengths and difficulties revealed in the report | Recommendations/programme show no links to individual's pattern of strengths and weaknesses |
| Recommendations specific and detailed | Recommendations vague and unspecific |
| Programme draws on individual's interests and needs; where a published programme is used, it is adapted to match individual needs | Heavy reliance on published materials (or on one published teaching programme) – programme not individual |
| Programme provides ideas for multisensory teaching | Heavy reliance on worksheets rather than multisensory methods |
| Programme matches teaching objectives to relevant curricular needs | Programme takes no account of curricular needs |

| Good practice | Weak practice |
|---|---|
| Programme appropriate for age and stage in both objectives and methods | Programme not age-appropriate |
| Both long-term and short-term targets for learning are outlined and supported by recommendations for method and pace | Programme does not define teaching/learning objectives |

## Overall style

| Good practice | Weak practice |
|---|---|
| Clear, plain English, jargon-free | Obscure, uses jargon |
| Language appropriate for audience | Language inappropriate for audience |
| Succinct, to the point | Wordy, rambling |
| Uses terminology correctly | Misuses terminology |
| Explains any 'technical' vocabulary | Uses terminology which would not be widely understood without any explanation |
| Acceptable standard of written English | Grammatical and/or spelling mistakes, colloquial style |
| Non-patronising style | 'Talks down' to the reader |
| Well formatted, accessible, appropriate font | Difficult to read, inaccessible |
| Well prioritised – main points and/or conclusions stand out clearly in the text | Difficult to locate main points |
| Teaching programme clearly separated from rest of report | Teaching programme mixed in with other information |

# 13.4 **Questionnaires**     Gill Backhouse

In order to gather the background information needed before an assessment, you will need to design questionnaires suitable for your own working context. If you work in schools, personal information about developmental history will be obtained from parents/carers. This information will generally be provided by learners in the 16+ age group themselves, so a questionnaire should be designed with this in mind. In both cases a second questionnaire is required to obtain information from teachers or tutors. This should be addressed to the Head Teacher or Head of Year in a secondary school. Their permission is normally required before relevant staff are involved in providing confidential information about pupils.

A large '**Confidential**' at the beginning provides reassurance that you will treat personal information with respect. Remember to put your contact details (full name and qualifications, position, work address, telephone and fax numbers; e-mail address) at the top and say why you need the information and by when. Include a box for the person completing the questionnaire to print and then sign his/her name, position (if relevant), telephone number and e-mail address.

You should explain that the assessment will focus on language and literacy skills, whether they are at the expected level and, if not, seek to establish the nature of and reason for difficulties. Your introduction to learners/parents should emphasise that in order to be valid, assessment results need to be viewed in the context of the developmental history. The introduction for teachers/tutors should make it clear that you regard your role as supportive of theirs; you need the knowledge they have regarding the learner in his normal educational setting; and will collaborate with them when considering any recommendations for learning support.

Questionnaires should be clearly set out and printed (Arial 12 point font is recommended), with plenty of room for responses. Many people now prefer to use a computer, so, if possible, make the forms available electronically. The form for school or college should be as brief as possible, so that busy teachers are not alienated.

Remember that the learner or his parents may well have language/literacy difficulties and so keep their form as brief as possible too. Questions should be phrased succinctly in single clauses. Respondents can either be invited to underline answers (Yes/No, or Yes/Perhaps/No), if appropriate, and/or space left for them to respond in their own words.

The issues to be covered are set out below. They cover areas of particular interest from the SpLD point of view, but also more general probes. Your aim is to obtain an holistic picture of the learner. *You are not trying to prove he is, or is not, dyslexic at this point!*

## *Parents/carers and learners*

- **Family background** including first language: history of language/literacy difficulties in relatives.

- **Physical development:** birth and early years; 'milestones' (sitting up, crawling, walking); ease with which self-care skills attained (feeding, dressing); fine and gross motor skills, coordination.

- **Health:** serious illnesses and accidents; chronic/recurring conditions (allergies, colds, ear infections). Hearing and vision.

- **Language and speech:** development pre-school; current communication skills; SLT referrals/treatment.

- **Temperament:** placid↔highly-strung, self-contained↔outgoing.

- **Interests:** sports, active-outdoor pursuits, practical activities, computer games, books, music, TV, socialising, etc.

- **Education:** schools/colleges/courses attended; adaptation to school and progress with basic skills; learning support (in school or privately arranged); study skills competence (for older learners); qualifications achieved.

- **Reason for referral**

- **Previous assessments:** ask for copies.

## *Teachers/tutors*

- Learner's attendance record; social adjustment and behaviour; confidence and self-esteem.

- Attitude to work, attention and ability to concentrate.

- Language skills: learner's ability to express himself, respond to instructions and questions.

- Strengths and weaknesses: different subjects; oral cf. written work.

- Level of attainments in basic skills: test and/or exam results.

- SENs recognised: learning support provision; access arrangements.

- Other relevant information.

- Specific concerns.

# 13.5  Assessment resources

| Name of Test | Date | Authors | Publishers | Age Range |
|---|---|---|---|---|
| Access Reading Test | 2006 | McCarty, C. and Crumpler, M | Hodder and Stoughton | 7–20+ years range |
| Adult Reading Test | 2004 | Brooks, P., Everatt, J. and Fidler, R. | Roehampton, University of Surrey | Adult age range |
| Assessment Battery for Dyslexia Screening in Higher Education | 2004 | York Adult Assessment | Dyslexia Institute and Centre for Reading and Language, University of York | Adult age range |
| Assessment of Handwriting Speed | 2001 | Allcock, P. | Patoss | Year 7–Year 11 |
| Beery Buktenica Visual Motor Integration Test (VMI), 5th edition | 2004 | Beery, K. E., Buktenica, N. A. and Beery, N. A. | Ann Arbor | 2–18 years |
| British Picture Vocabulary Scale (BPVS), 2nd edition | 1997 | Dunn, L. and Dunn, L. | NFER-Nelson | 3 years–15 years 8 months |
| Checking Individual Progression in Phonics (ChiPPs) | 2001 | Palmer, S. and Reason, R. | NFER-Nelson | 6–7 years |
| Comprehensive Test of Phonological Processing (CToPP) | 1999 | Wagner, R., Torgeson, J. and Rashotte, C. | Pro-Ed | 5 years–24 years 11 months |
| Diagnostic Reading Analysis | 2004 | Crumpler, M. and McCarty, C. | Hodder and Stoughton | 7–16 years |
| Digit Memory Test | Rev. 2002 | Ridsdale, J. and Turner, M. | Dyslexia Institute website | 6 years–adult |

| Name of Test | Date | Authors | Publishers | Age Range |
|---|---|---|---|---|
| Dyscalculia Screener | 2004 | Butterworth, B. | NFER-Nelson | 6–14 years |
| Dyslexia Adult Screening Test (DAST) | 1998 | Fawcett, A. and Nicholson, R. | The Psychological Corporation (now Harcourt Assessment) | 16 years 5 months+ |
| Dyslexia Early Screening Test, 2nd edition | 2004 | Fawcett, A. and Nicholson, R. | The Psychological Corporation (now Harcourt Assessment) | 4 years 6 months–6 years 5 months |
| Dyslexia Screener | 2004 | Smith, P. and Turner, M. | NFER-Nelson | 5–16 years |
| Dyslexia Screening Test (DST) | 1996 | Fawcett, A. and Nicholson, R. | Psychological Corporation (now Harcourt Assessment) | 6 years 6 months–16 years 5 months |
| Edinburgh Reading Tests 1–4 | 2002 | Educational Assessment Unit, University of Edinburgh | Hodder and Stoughton | Four tests cover age range 7–17 years |
| Graded Arithmetic-Mathematics Test | 1998 | Vernon, P. E. and Miller, K. M. | Hodder and Stoughton | 5–12 years |
| Graded Word Reading Test | 1983 | The Macmillan Test Unit | NFER-Nelson | 6–14 years |
| Graded Word Spelling Test | 1977, 2006 | Vernon, P. E. | Hodder and Stoughton | 5–18+ years |
| Gray Oral Reading Tests (GORT-4) | 2000 | Wiederholt, J. Lee and Bryant, B. R. | Pro-Ed Inc | 6 years–18 years 11 months |
| Gray Silent Reading Test (GSRT) | 2002 | Wiederholt, J. Lee and Blalock, G. | Pro-Ed Inc | 7–25 years |
| Helen Arkell Word Spelling Test (HAST) | 1998 | | Helen Arkell Dyslexia Centre | 5–17+ years |

| Name of Test | Date | Authors | Publishers | Age Range |
|---|---|---|---|---|
| Individual Reading Analysis | 1989 | Vincent, D. and de la Mare, M. | NFER-Nelson | 5 years 6 months–11 years 2 months |
| LADs Adult Dyslexia Screening | 2004 | | Lucid Research | 16+ years |
| LASS Junior | 2003 | | Lucid Research | 8–11 years |
| LASS Secondary | 2003 | | Lucid Research | 11–15 years |
| Lucid CoPs | 2003 | | Lucid Research | 4–8 years |
| Mathematics Competency Test | 1995 | Vernon, P. E., Miller, K. M. and Izard, J. F. | Hodder and Stoughton | 11 years–adult |
| Morrisby Manual Dexterity Test | 1991 | | The Morrisby Organisation | 10+ years |
| Motor Screening Test | 1996 | From *Developmental Dyspraxia* by Madeleine Portwood | David Fulton Publishers | 7+ years |
| Movement Assessment Battery for Children (Movement ABC) | 1992 | Henderson, S. E. and Sugden, D. A. | Psychological Corporation (now Harcourt Assessment) | 6–9+ years |
| Naglieri Nonverbal Ability Test | 2002, 1997 | Naglieri, J. A. | Psychological Corporation (now Harcourt Assessment) | 5–17 years |
| Neale Analysis of Reading Ability–2nd Revised British Edition | 1989 | Neale, M. D. | NFER-Nelson | 6 years–12 years 11 months |
| New Reading Analysis | 1985 | Vincent, D. and de la Mare, M. | NFER-Nelson | 7 years 5 months–13 years |

| Name of Test | Date | Authors | Publishers | Age Range |
|---|---|---|---|---|
| Nonword Reading Test | 2004 | Crumpler, M. and McCarty, C. | Hodder and Stoughton | 6–16+ years |
| Parallel Spelling Tests | 1983 | Young, D. | Hodder and Stoughton | 6–15 years |
| Peabody Picture Vocabulary Test III | 1997 | Dunn, L. and Dunn, L. | American Guidance Service | 2 years 6 months–90+ years |
| Perin Spoonerism Test | 1983 | Perin, D. | In *British Journal of Psychology*, 74, 129–44, 1983 (available from Dyslexia Institute website) | 14–15 years |
| Phonological Abilities Test (PAT) | 1997 | Muter, V., Hulme, C. and Snowling, M. J. | Psychological Corporation (now Harcourt Assessment) | 5–7 years |
| Phonological Assessment Battery (PhAB) | 1997 | Fredrickson, N., Frith, U. and Reason, R. | NFER-Nelson | 6–14 years |
| Pre-school and Primary Inventory of Phonological Awareness (PIPA) | 2000 | Dodd, B., Crosbie, S., McIntosh, B., Teitzel, T. and Ozanne, A. | Psychological Corporation (now Harcourt Assessment) | 3 years–6 years 11 months |
| Ravens Coloured Progressive Matrices (RCPM) | 1988 | Raven, J. C., Court, J. H., Raven, J. | Oxford Psychologists Press | 5–11 years |
| Ravens Standard Progressive Matrices (RSPM) | 1988 | Raven, J. C., Court, J. H., Raven, J. | Oxford Psychologists Press | 6+ years–adult |
| Sentence Completion Test | 1995 | Hedderly, R. | Dyslexia Institute website | 9–18 years |
| Sound Linkage | 2000 | Hatcher, P. | Whurr | 7+ years |

| Name of Test | Date | Authors | Publishers | Age Range |
|---|---|---|---|---|
| Spadafore Diagnostic Reading Test (SDRT) | 1983 | Spadafore, G. J. | Academic Therapy Publications, California | 6 years–adult |
| Spatial Reasoning Tests | | Smith, P. and Lord, T. R. | NFER-Nelson | 6–14 years |
| Symbol Digit Modalities Test (SDMT) | 1982 | Smith, A. | Western Psychological Services | 8–17 years |
| Test of Word Reading Efficiency (TOWRE) | 1999 | Torgesen, J. K., Wagner, R. K. and Rashotte, C. A. | Pro-Ed (available in UK from Harcourt Assessment) | 6–24 years 11 months |
| Vernon-Warden Reading Test | 1995 | Hedderly, R. | In *Dyslexia Review*, 7, 3 Autumn 1995. Available from Dyslexia Institute website | 8 years–adult |
| Wide Range Achievement Test III (WRAT–3) Reading, Spelling and Arithmetic | 1993 | Wilkinson, G. S. | Wide Range Inc. (available in UK from Harcourt Assessment) | 5–75 years |
| Wide Range Achievement Test III–Expanded Edition (WRAT–E) | 2001 | Wilkinson, G. S. | Wide Range Inc. (available in UK from Harcourt Assessment) | 5–18 years |
| Wide Range Assessment of Memory and Learning 2nd edition (WRAML–2) | 2003 | Sheslow, D. and Adams, W. | Wide Range Inc | 5–90 years |

| Name of Test | Date | Authors | Publishers | Age Range |
|---|---|---|---|---|
| Wide Range Intelligence Test (WRIT) | 2000 | Glutting, J., Adams, W. and Sheslow, D. | Wide Range Inc (available from Dyslexia Institute) | 4–84 years |
| Word Recognition and Phonic Skills (WRaPS) | 2003 | Moseley, D. | Hodder and Stoughton | 4 years 6 months–9 years |
| Wordchains | 1999 | Guron, L. M. | NFER-Nelson | 7 years to adult |
| Working Memory Test Battery for Children (WMTB-C) | 2001 | Pickering, S. and Gathercole, S. | Psychological Corporation (now Harcourt Assessment) | 5–15 years |
| York Adult Assessment Battery | See *Assessment Battery for Dyslexia Screening in Higher Education*, above | | | |

# 13.6  References

**(See section 13.5 for references to specific tests and assessments)**

Alston, J. (1995) *Assessing and Promoting Writing Skills*, NASEN.

Alston, J. and Taylor, J. (1992) *Handwriting Helpline*, Dextral Books.

APA (1994). *Diagnostic and Statistical Manual of Mental Disorders*, fourth edition, Washington, DC: American Psychiatric Association.

Ausubel, D. P. (1968) *Educational Psychology, A Cognitive View*, New York: Holt, Rinehart and Winston.

Backhouse, G. (2000) *Providing For Candidates With Special Assessment Needs During GCE (A-level), VCE, GCSE and GNVQ: A Practical Guide*, Evesham: Patoss.

Backhouse, G., Dolman, E., and Read, C. (2004) *Dyslexia: Assessing the Need for Access Arrangements: the Patoss Guide*, second edition, Evesham: Patoss in association with the Joint Council for Qualifications.

Baddeley, A. D. (1986) *Working Memory*, Oxford: Oxford University Press.

Baddeley A. D. and Hitch, G. (1974) 'Working memory', in G. A. Bower (ed.) *The Psychology of Learning and Motivation*, Vol. 8, New York: Academic Press.

Barnett, A. L. and Henderson, S. E. (2004) 'Assessment of Handwriting in Children with Development Coordination Disorder', in Sugden, D. A. and Chambers, M. E. (eds) *Children with Developmental Coordination Disorder*, London: Whurr.

Basic Skills Agency (2001) *Adult Literacy Core Curriculum*, London: BSA.

Beech, J. R. and Singleton, C. (1997) *The Psychological Assessment of Reading*, London: Routledge.

Booth, G. (1996) 'Principles of Assessment' in Reid, G. (ed.) *Dimensions of Dyslexia*, Vol. 1, Edinburgh: Moray House Publications.

BPS (1999) *Dyslexia, Literacy and Psychological Assessment*. Leicester: British Psychological Society.

BPS Psychological Testing Centre (2004) *Psychological Testing: A User's Guide*. Available online from www.psychtesting.org

Bristow, J., Cowley, P. and Daines, B. (1999) *Memory and Learning – A Practical Guide*, London: David Fulton.

Bryant, P. and Bradley, L. (1985) *Children's Reading Difficulties*, Oxford: Blackwell.

Butterworth, B. and Yeo, D. (2004) *Dyscalculia Guidance*, Windsor: NFER-Nelson.

Clay, M. (2000) *An Observational Study of Early Literacy Achievement*, second edition, Auckland: Heinemann.

DfEE (Department for Education and Employment) (1998) *The National Literacy Strategy Framework for teaching*, London: The Stationery Office.

DfEE (1999a) *The National Curriculum: Handbooks for Primary Teachers*, HMSO (www.nc.uk.net).

DfEE (1999b) *The National Curriculum: Handbooks for Secondary Teachers*, HMSO (www.nc.uk.net).

DfES (Department for Education and Skills) (2001) *Code of Practice for the Identification and Assessment of Special Educational Needs*, London: The Stationery Office.

DfES (2004a) *A Framework for Understanding Dyslexia*, DfES Publications.

DfES (2004b) *Every Child Matters*, DfES Publications.

DfES (2004c) *Removing Barriers to Achievement: The Government's SEN Strategy*, DfES Publications.

DRC (Disability Rights Commission) (2002a) *Disability Discrimination Act 1995 Part 4: Code of Practice for Providers of Post 16 Education and Related Services*, www.drc.gov.uk/thelaw/practice.asp

DRC (2002b) *Disability Discrimination Act 1995 Part 4: Code of Practice for Schools*, www.drc.gov.uk/thelaw/practice.asp

DRC (2004) Information from the DRC's website, August 2004 (http://www.drc-gb.org/).

Ehri, L. C. (2002) 'Phases of acquisition in learning to read words and implications for teaching' in *Learning and Teaching Reading British. Journal of Educational Psychology. Monograph Series II: Psychological Aspects of Education – Current Trends. No.1.*

Foulkes, G. (2003) Speech to ACCAC: Access to Assessment and Qualifications Conference: Cardiff, 21 June 2003 (www.accac.org.uk).

Freeman, J. (2000) 'Literacy, Flexible Thinking and Underachievement', in Montgomery, D. (ed.) *Able Underachievers*, London: Whurr.

Frith, U. (1985) 'Beneath the Surface of Developmental Dyslexia', in Patterson, K., Coltheart, M. and Marshall, J. (eds) *Surface Dyslexia*, London: Routledge and Kegan Paul.

Goswami, U. and Bryant, P. (1990) *Phonological Skills and Learning to Read*, London: Lawrence Erlbaum.

Gough, B. and Tunmer, E. (1986) 'Decoding, reading and reading disability', *Remedial and Special Education*, 7, 6–10.

Goulandris, N. (2002) *Dyslexia: Cross-Linguistic Comparisons*, London: Whurr.

Gross, J. (2002) *Special Educational Needs in the Primary School*, third edition, Buckingham: Open University Press.

Handy, C. (2000) *The Age of Unreason*, Arrow Business Books.

Hatcher, P. J. (2000) *Sound Linkage: An Integrated Programme for Overcoming Reading Difficulties* (second edition), London: Whurr.

Hatcher, J., Snowling, M. J. and Griffiths, Y. M. (2002) 'Cognitive assessment of dyslexic students in higher education', *British Journal of Educational Psychology*, *72*, 119–33 (reprints available from: Department of Psychology, University of York, York YO10 5DD).

Hook, P. and Jones, S. (2002) 'The importance of automaticity and fluency for efficient reading comprehension', *Perspectives*, *28*, 1, 9–14.

Howley, M. and Kime, S. (2003) in Tilstone, C. and Rose, R. (eds) *Strategies to Promote Inclusive Practice*, London: Routledge Falmer.

Johnson Levine, K. (1991) *Fine Motor Dysfunction: Therapeutic Strategies in the Classroom*, Oxford: Harcourt.

Johnson, M., Peer, L. and Lee, R. (2001) 'Pre-school children and dyslexia: policy, identification and intervention', in Fawcett, A. (ed.) *Dyslexia Theory and Good Practice*, London : Whurr.

Joint Committee on the Draft Disability Discrimination Bill (2004) *First Report Chapter 12: Examining Bodies and Standard Setting Agencies*. *http://www.publications.parliament.uk/pa/jt200304/jtselect/jtdisab/82/8215.htm*

Layton, L., Deeny, K. and Upton, G. (1997) *Sound Practice – Phonological Awareness in the Classroom*, London: David Fulton.

Levine, M. (1994) *Educational Care – a System for Understanding and Helping Children With Learning Problems at Home and in School*, Cambridge, Massachusetts: Educators Publishing Service.

Long, M. (2004) Fry Readability Graph (online) available from: www.psych-ed.org/ (accessed 11 September 2004).

Lundberg, I. and Hoien, T. (2001) 'Dyslexia and Phonology', in Fawcett, A. (ed.) *Dyslexia Theory and Good Practice*, London: Whurr.

Morton, J. and Frith, U. (1995). *Dyslexia, Literacy and Psychological Assessment*. A Report of a Working Party of the Division of Educational and Child Psychology of the British Psychological Society (1999), Leicester: British Psychological Society.

Muter, V. (2003) *Early Reading Development and Dyslexia*, London: Whurr.

Paulesu, E., Frith, U., Snowling, M. J. et al (1996) 'Is developmental dyslexia a disconnection syndrome? Evidence from PET scanning', *Brain*, *119*, 143–57.

Pinney, A. (2004) *Reducing Reliance on Statements: An Investigation into Local Authority Practice and Outcomes Research Brief RB508*, DfES Publications.

Pollock, J. and Waller, E. (1994) *Day-to-Day Dyslexia in the Classroom*, London: Routledge.

Portwood, M. (1996) *Developmental Dyspraxia*, London: David Fulton.

QCA (2003) *Foundation Stage Profile Handbook*, London: Qualification and Curriculum Authority.

QCA (2000) *Curriculum Guidance for the Foundation Stage*, London: Qualifications and Curriculum Authority.

Reason, R. (2004) In *Dyslexia – A Landmark High Court Judgement*, online: www.bps.org.uk

Reid, G. and Wearmouth, J. (2002) 'Issues for Assessment and Planning of Teaching and Learning', in *Dyslexia and Literacy: Theory and Practice*, Wiley.

Rice, M. and Brooks, G. (2004) *Developmental dyslexia in adults: a research review*, London: National Research and Development Centre for adult literacy and numeracy.

Saunders, K. and White, A. (2002) *How Dyslexics Learn, Grasping the Nettle*, Evesham: Patoss.

Schools Examination and Assessment Council (SEAC) (1992) *Interim Report on Research Project: Special Educational Needs and the GCSE*. Commissioned from the Centre for Assessment Studies, University of Bristol.

Seidenberg, M. S. (2002) 'Using connectionist models to understand reading and dyslexia', in Learning and Teaching Reading, *British Journal of Educational Psychology. Monograph Series II: Psychological Aspects of Education – Current Trends. No.1.*

Snowling, M. J. (2000) *Dyslexia*, second edition, Oxford: Blackwell.

Special Educational Needs Code of Practice (2001) DfES Publications.

Spooner, A. L. R., Baddeley, A. and Gathercole, S. E. (2004) 'Can reading accuracy and comprehension be separated in the Neale Analysis of Reading Ability?', *British Journal of Educational Psychology*, 74, 187–204.

Stackhouse J. and Wells, B. (1997) *Children's Speech and Literacy Difficulties: Book 1: A Psycholinguistic Framework*, London: Whurr.

Stackhouse, J. and Wells, B. (2001) *Children's Speech and Literacy Difficulties: Book 2*, London: Whurr.

Taylor, J. (1999) 'Pupils' Self-Evaluation as an Aid to Teaching Handwriting', in: Snowling, M. J. and Thompson, M. *Dyslexia: Integrating Theory and Practice*, London: Whurr.

Topping, K. (1995) *Paired Reading, Writing and Spelling*, London: Cassell.

Turner, M. (1997) *Psychological Assessment of Dyslexia*, London: Whurr.

Vellutino, F., Pruzek, R., Steger, J. and Meshoulam, U. (1973) 'Immediate visual recall in poor readers as a function of orthographic-linguistic familiarity', *Cortex*, *9*, 368–84.

West, T. G. (1991) *In the Mind's Eye: Visual Thinkers, Gifted People with Learning Difficulties, Computer Images and the Ironies of Creativity*, London: Prometheus Books.

Wood, J., Wright, J., Stackhouse, J. (2000) *Language and Literacy: Joining Together*, Reading: British Dyslexia Association/Afasic.

# 13.7  Useful websites and contacts

| | |
|---|---|
| Adult Dyslexia Organisation (ADO) | www.futurenet.co.uk/charity/ado/adomenu/adomenu.htm |
| Advisory Centre for Education (ACE) | www.ace-ed.org.uk |
| Association For All Speech-Impaired Children | www.afasic.org.uk |
| Association of Dyslexia Specialists in Higher Education (ADSHE) | www.adshe.org.uk  www.natdisteam.ac.uk |
| Attention Deficit Disorder Information Services | www.addiss.co.uk |
| Basic Skills Agency | www.basic-skills.co.uk |
| Bridging the Gap; A guide to the Disabled Students Allowances (DSAs) in Higher Education (tel: 0800 731 9133) | www.dfes.gov.uk/studentsupport |
| British Association of Occupational Therapists; College of Occupational Therapists | www.cot.co.uk |
| British Dyslexia Association | www.bda-dyslexia.org.uk |
| British Psychological Society | www.bps.org.uk |
| British Society of Audiology | www.thebsa.org.uk |
| Cerium Visual Technologies (supplies tinted overlays and can provide a list of colorimetry specialists in local areas) | www.ceriumvistech.co.uk |
| Chartered Society of Physiotherapy | www.csp.org.uk |
| Connexions | www.connexions.gov.uk |
| Correct Punctuation | www.correctpunctuation.co.uk |
| Department for Education and Skills | www.dfes.gov.uk |
| Disability Discrimination Act (DDA) | www.disability.gov.uk/dda |
| Disability Rights Commission (DRC) | www.drc-gb.org |
| Disability Rights Task Force | www.disability.gov.uk |
| Dyslexia Institute (now Dyslexia Action) | www.dyslexia-inst.org.uk |
| Dyslexia Teaching and Adult Training Centre | dyslexiateacher@tiscali.co.uk |
| Dyspraxia Foundation | www.dyspraxiafoundation.org.uk |
| Dyspraxia Support: Developmental Adult Neuro-Diversity Association | www.danda.org.uk |
| Handwriting Interest Group | www.nha-handwriting.org.uk |

| | |
|---|---|
| Her Majesty's Stationery Office | www.hmso.gov.uk |
| Higher Education Funding Council for England | www.hefce.ac.uk |
| iANSYST | www.dyslexic.com |
| Institute of Education, University of London | www.ioe.ac.uk |
| Institute of Optometry | www.ioo.org.uk |
| Joint Council for Qualifications | www.jcq.org.uk |
| Learning and Skills Council | www.lsc.gov.uk |
| Learning and Skills Development Agency | www.lsda.org.uk |
| National Association for Special Educational Needs (NASEN) | www.nasen.org.uk |
| National Association of Disability Officers (NADO) | www.nado.org.uk |
| National Disability Team. Supporting Disabled Students in Higher Education | www.natdisteam.ac.uk |
| Office for Advice, Assistance, Support and Information on Special Needs | www.oaasis.co.uk |
| Patoss: The Professional Association of Teachers of Students with Specific Learning Difficulties | www.patoss-dyslexia.org |
| Qualifications and Curriculum Authority | www.qca.org.uk |
| Quality Assurance Agency for Higher Education | www.qaa.ac.uk |
| Royal College of Speech and Language Therapists | www.rcslt.org |
| SKILL National Bureau for Students with Disabilities | www.skill.org.uk |
| Support for Learning | www.support4learning.org.uk |
| Teacher Training Agency | www.canteach.gov.uk |
| The Stationery Office (TSO) | www.tso-online.co.uk |
| World of Dyslexia Ltd | www.dyslexia-adults.com; www.dyslexia-college.com |

## Publishers' websites

| | |
|---|---|
| David Fulton Publishers | www.fultonpublishers.co.uk |
| Heinemann Educational | www.heinemann.co.uk |

| | |
|---|---|
| Hodder and Stoughton/Hodder Murray | www.hoddereducation.co.uk; www.hoddertests.co.uk |
| Lucid Research Ltd | www.lucid-research.com |
| Morrisby Organisation | www.morrisby.com |
| NFER-Nelson | www.nfer-nelson.co.uk |
| Oxford Psychologists Press | www.opp.co.uk |
| Pro-ed | www.proedinc.com |
| Psychological Corporation (now Harcourt Assessment) | www.harcourtassessment.com |
| SENTER AMS Educational | www.senter.co.uk |
| Whurr Publishers | www.whurr.co.uk |

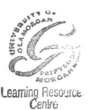